Dancing with Arthritis
At
Arthur Murray

H.B. Jones

Dancing with Arthritis at Arthur Murray- H.B. Jones
Copyright © 2019 H.B. Jones

For information contact :
Barney Jones at 86andmore@gmail.com

Why I began dance lessons at age 86
Young or old, you too can learn to dance

Dedication

I dedicate this book to the entire staff and all the students at the Arthur Murray Center in Folsom, California.

Acknowledgements

I would like to thank Kate Gonzalez, owner, director and teacher at the Folsom Arthur Murray franchise for providing me with the technical information of Arthur Murray operations, and also for her professional and friendly management of this local dance center.

I also wish to thank those students who graciously shared their dance experiences along with me in this book.

Lastly, I am indebted to all my fellow students for their friendship, their support and their amiable acceptance of such an old dog in their midst. They and our teachers make me feel like this is a second home.

Author's Note

Neither my guest writers nor I have received any financial remuneration, favors or promises from any Arthur Murray Franchise or Corporation. We are simply relating the truth of our experiences at this dance center.

Chapter One
Why Should We Dance?

It's not that I haven't ever danced before, but back in the day where I grew up we didn't worry about doing any stinkin' steps or fancy footwork, so it wasn't real dancing.

In high school it was just an excuse to hold a girl close while shuffling around and trying to think of something clever to say. That was the only time I was allowed to take ahold of a girl and bring her close to me. I thought it was funny that if I held a girl that close to me in the school hallway, the school authorities would have practically accused me of a sex crime, but if I were doing it on the dance floor, they thought it was cute.

I was always hoping for a real slow tune so I had an excuse to tighten the embrace and get even closer.

♫ *Put another nickel in, in the nickelodeon, all I want is you….♫..closer, my dear, come closer…*

Yeah, that was me in my early teens. Didn't get much better in my late teens.

But let me clarify that my reasons for wanting to dance now are *completely different*.

Why does it take dynamite or a stiff drink to motivate average Americans to get off their rear and onto a dance floor? My students in Spanish classes resisted dancing or singing of any kind, insisting, "It's not cool." Many older Americans claim they "can't dance" or "have two left feet" and won't even try. Or they resort to the untutored *Freestyle* which can sometimes lead to bizarre gyrations, arm thrusts, and neck pops, which may be creative, but not always controlled or graceful.

I think this attitude simply reveals that dancing is not part of our national culture, like in Cuba, where it's a way of life; there, dancing is as natural as eating and walking. Meanwhile we're sitting it out and they're having the fun.

Running is another activity that is loved by some and avoided by others. In his book *Born to Run,* Christopher McDougall cites an ultra-distance running coach who made the surprising conclusion that the Tarahumara Indians of Mexico win so many races because of their orientation of kindness toward others, as well as their culture and passion for running.

The same may be said of dancing. Whether it's a passion or a pastime, it's fun. When we're having fun, we are upbeat and feel kindly towards the other folks there who are enjoying themselves in the same way.

Dancing is a very social activity. In a ballroom or dancehall the energy is positive and congenial. The Arthur Murray dance center where I go is one of the happiest places on our troubled planet.

Have you put on a few extra pounds lately? Another benefit from dancing is the physical exercise. It's also a way to make new friends, and spend leisure time productively and joyfully.

Do you feel your joints getting a bit stiff? The best treatment for an arthritic joint is . . . *MOVEMENT*.

Do you have that middle-age slump? Dancing is also a motivator to improve your posture, whether you're middle-aged, a spring chicken, or an old rooster.

Are you starting to forget words or names? One of the most vital benefits of dance lessons is the challenge to the brain, which can help to prevent Alzheimer's disease.

What are you waiting for?

Chapter Two
Early Dance Dramas

It wasn't until my mid twenties that I did any real dancing, and even then I didn't do it right. I was a college student in Denver, Colorado and happened upon a kind of a rough joint called the *Blue Blaze*. The music they were playing affected me as though an electric currant had ahold of me, demanding that I bounce to the beat.

It was polka music, but at that time I didn't know a polka from an Irish Jig. All I knew was that the rhythm took possession of my soul and body. I couldn't sit still; I had to get up and hop around.

Most of the crowd there was of German extraction, and some didn't even speak English. They regarded me with an air of amusement mixed with resentment. I was an outsider who was trying to dance to *their* music with *their* girls in *their* hangout.

However, that music so captivated me that I came back with a few friends of my own. But watching those German immigrants dance confused me. Many of them were not dancing the same polka step as the others. Instead they were doing something I learned was called the *Dutch Hop*. I learned later that it was a tradition the *Volga Germans* in Russia brought over from the old country. I tried to imitate them and ended up doing a half-assed and inept hybrid of both styles, and not a good imitation of either. But it still kept our spirits high and eventually I learned the traditional polka hop.

As long as I was in Denver, I did my best to infect as many of my friends as possible with the polka bug, especially potential dance partners.

But then my school term was over and I continued my studies in another country, met a girl, got married, started working, and raised a family. The polka had drifted far away from my mind...but not my soul.

One evening many years later in the town where my family and I had settled, I was driving by a community center and heard the resonant strains of a polka. My former musical senses jumped back to life. It was a bona fide polka club, called the *Polka Boosters*. I even got my wife, raised as a Southern Baptist, enthused, and we danced there often. Much later, when I found myself lonely and single again, I mustard up some friends to enjoy this dance with me; and the bug bit them too.

But eventually I got mountain fever, and left the flatlands, the polka and all dancing behind for a lengthy hiatus. How long would it last this time?

Dancing in The Sixties

I experienced two other dance episodes, both very brief, but each one extremely memorable. I have revisited these two interludes in my mind many times since.

These mini adventures took place during the zany sixties, when a *gas* meant a good time, and *going ape* was to act crazy, and when someone was *bad,* it meant he was really good. *Flower Power* was in vogue with the slogan *it it feels good, do it.*

When couples danced, they didn't touch, and there was no frame or steps to stifle the creativity. This phenomenon was called *freestyle and* was undisciplined and occasionally frenzied.

Some could carry it off without making complete asses of themselves. But many, like the Elaine character on the TV program *Seinfeld,* looked contorted, jabbing a leg out like she's kicking butt, and throwing her head back so violently that it looked like it could break her neck. She thought she looked bad (awesome), but those watching were just embarrassed for her.

And some of the guys were even worse. I remember watching this young cat who was showing off his freestyle skills. He raised one knee up higher than his waist, balancing on the other foot, then he spun crazily around, almost losing his balance, waived both hands high in the air, then flung one hand down like he was trying to shake off a glob of mud, or something worse, then he stuck one foot out in front, did a little hop, then squatted down low, then came up and started gyrating his hips and torso, trying to look sexy, but instead appeared to be having a seizure. He thought he looked bad—meaning great. How ridiculous can you get! I could never be that uninhibited, nor did I want to be!

This dance style was not limited to our country, as I found out in 1965 when I went abroad at age thirty-six. I had been awarded a government grant along with other Spanish teachers of both genders, to spend the summer in Burgos, Spain, to study the language and culture. Even though I was married, I couldn't help but notice that many of the female teachers were young, attractive, single and out for a good time during their leisure hours.

There was one Saturday night that comes to mind. We had been studying for several weeks when I found myself galavanting in Madrid with a couple of my male classmates. Our sponsors had taken us to the big city for a cultural tour. The last night there they had scheduled a dinner and later we were all to go to a night club for some dancing.

But before the dance scene, these two characters, my buddies, insisted that before going to the night club where the rest of our classmates were, we should cut out to "see some of Madrid's hotspots."

After the mandatory drink at each of the establishments that we were checking out, our live-it-up-pub-hopping craze was appeased and replaced by Saturday night fever, so we joined our classmates at the nightclub where they were dancing.

With my alcohol intolerance for more than two beers, I knew I had to sweat out the evil brew or I might lose that good dinner I had ingested earlier. And how was I going to work out those toxins? *FREESTYLE* dancing, as that is what everyone there was doing. One thing I didn't have to worry abut was my usual inhibitions, because in my current state they were non-existent!

So, since I knew no better, I unwisely followed the one terrible example I had previously witnessed. I really *went ape,* according to my classmate's description. I starting dancing by raising one knee up higher than my waist, balancing on one foot, then I spun crazily around, almost losing my balance, waved both hands high in the air, then flung one hand down like I was trying to shake off a glob of mud, or something worse, then stuck one foot our in front, did a little hop, then squatted down low and came up and started gyrating my hips and torso, trying to look sexy, but instead probably looked more like I was having a seizure. I was bad—meaning really awful. But I thought, *man, this is a gas!*

I think my pretty partners were happy too; anyway, every time I saw them looking at me while we were dancing, they were laughing.

The next morning we loaded the bus for our return to Burgos. I was not sick, but neither was I feeling real chipper. I laid my head back on the seat and closed my eyes. Then I became aware that one of the cutie pies had left her seat by her boyfriend to come sit by me. She put her hand on my forehead, then placed a cool, damp cloth on it.

"We decided you probably needed some TLC this morning" she whispered. I didn't argue, but I wondered why they thought I needed any special care.

Nowadays there are still many who resort to freestyle dancing, rather than learn steps and dance with a partner, actually holding on to them, heaven forbid. Well, it still is dancing, and they're moving to music, so it's not all bad. Still it seems to me to be kind of lazy, the easiest way out, the second best, lacking any real challenge. Besides, the brain needs exercise too— learning dance patterns helps ward off Alzheimers.

I had friendships with some of the pretty young teachers in Spain, but unlike several of my male, married colleagues, I managed to avoid any intimate liaison with any of them. After all, I was a married man with a family. Avoiding a fling wasn't any great accomplishment because I have never been much of a babe magnet anyway.

But that was before I met Manuel's cousin. Manuel was my roommate and some of his family traveling in Europe then had come to visit him. Manuel invited me and a couple of female classmates to have dinner with him and his family to celebrate his birthday.

I was sitting across from Mariana, Manuel's gorgeous cousin. She was very easy to look at, so what the heck, that's what I did. With her smooth, delicate white facial skin, and pleasing features I judged her to be about nineteen, but her bearing seemed more mature. And while we chatted I learned that she was a fairly sophisticated twenty-six year old.

Mariana was about five foot one, slender, but had a mature figure that was nicely sculpted in a very feminine way. I found her to be well spoken, interesting, educated and quite . . . companionable. Our delightful conversation was flowing as freely as the champagne, which the waiter kept pouring. But I was too focused on this young woman to over indulge this night. The ambience between us felt warm, and along with a couple of subtle innuendos, our eyes met, and they were saying more, searching and suggesting.

From the restaurant we went to a dance sponsored by the host of this overseas program. Mariana and I were dancing a slow one and I held her very close. She was so deliciously petite that we fit together perfectly. I felt very . . . comfortable to be in this intimate embrace, floating on a fair weather cloud. My mind traveled back in time. This is what I used to try to go for when I was in my teens, I thought. My God, what am I doing?

Then she whispered softly in my ear: "I don't understand these guys." I knew she was talking about my male colleagues. "Clarence has been coming on to me," she said, "and he's thirty-four, married and has two kids."

I sighed . . . then I swallowed and said, "Well, I'm thirty-six, married and have four kids."

She looked up at me, her face drawn and her jaw dropped. She slowly backed out of our intimate embrace. The music stopped. The spell was broken. That was our last dance.

I had been hitchhiking on a cloud of romantic fantasy. I don't regret my ride in this brief but fantastic escapade in an otherworldly realm; neither do I regret my self-imposed descent back to my reality on Earth. But I will always remember that last dance.

Ah yes—there is such a thing as dancing for romance. We have all done that at some time, haven't we? Tender memories, exalted passions, but sometimes broken hearts?

♫Those were the days my friend, We thought they'd never end,We'd sing and dance forever and a day ♪

For me at this stage of life, I view dancing as a productive pastime, and a way to breakaway from the usual geriatric day-to-day tedium. For me dancing is a discipline, albeit a happy and satisfying one, as I mix with my friendly fellow students.

But bless all these young folks who look at dancing as a purely romantic opportunity. Bless the older folks too, if they're similarly inclined.

Chapter Three
Country Dance And Mountaineering

The only other dancing I ever did (that is, if you consider those two previous episodes dancing) was a few minutes of *country swing*. It was actually a few weeks and it was fun, but after a big bunch of years away from it I remembered not one whit of it. The fact is, I stopped all dancing completely for many years.

What! Why? How could I do that after all this build up here?! It could only be because I was infused with another passion: *Mountaineering*. I had retired and moved to my favorite playground, what John Muir called the *Range of Light*, the *Sierra Nevada* mountains near beautiful Lake Tahoe. With friends, I was fully engrossed in hiking, climbing, and my favorite, *ski mountaineering*. In this challenging but delightful discipline you are skiing in the back country in ungroomed snow away from ski resorts and chair lifts. You climb up to the mountain top, one ski stride at a time, and you ski back down through whatever kind of snow that mother nature has left for you that day. This called for techniques that enabled you to turn in varied snow conditions. We used a Norwegian move called the *Telemark Turn*. This and especially the *Telemark Jump Turn* required a long learning curve.

So what does all this have to do with dancing? Two things: It taught me that with perseverance I could learn to do things that at first seemed impossible, like the *tele-jumpturn*— and later, complicated dance patterns.

The other point is that Telemarking in the back country is kind of like a mountain ballet. As my expert telemarker nephew Dave Jones says, "You're dancing with the mountain—but the mountain is the leader."

Moving to The Old Folks Home

When I moved back down to the flatlands from my beloved Sierra, due to old age and medical issues, I ended up in a senior community with a bunch of old folks. Old, yeah, like me. Except not exactly like me.

To avoid confusion I let them call me by my real name, Harvey, rather than my nickname, Barney, (from my middle name), which I had been known as for most of my life. I still go by Barney with old friends and acquaintances. I like the name Barney better, but besides the fact that legally Barney Jones doesn't exist, the name seems to be associated with a host of weird or unsavory characters.

Now that I was a flatlander, I had to find a replacement for my Sierra ski ballet. I needed an active pastime and a challenge. I had always been drawn to dance, even when I wasn't doing it myself. Now I wanted to do it instead of think about or watch it. And I still had fond memories of my meagre past dance experiences.

I met a lady in this old folk's home who said she used to polka. "Wow," I said, "I used to do the polka too, and I loved it."

She told me that there was going to be an *October Fest* here in our building soon with a live band. "They always play some polkas," she said. "Why don't you come? We'll show these folks what a polka looks like."

Did I even remember how to polka? It had been nigh onto twenty years since I'd done that caper, so I practiced it in my apartment. And just like the old adage about riding a bicycle, if you knew it once, it comes right back.

So I danced the polka and a few shuffles with the ladies, and then met a younger resident I'll call Sweetie Pie, and I danced some with her until she moved on.

The ladies here don't hop around like they did in their twenties, but they do have an abundance of spirit. On New Year's Eve I danced with a gussied up lady whom I didn't recognize at first because she wasn't using her cane or walker. "I have braces on both knees," she said and she was ready to *shake her booty*.

At one point during a fast piece, I asked if her knees were all right. "I don't give a damn," she said, "It's New Year's Eve and my birthday, and I'm having a blast!"

Most of the ladies here, and sometimes men, who are still somewhat ambulatory, like to get out and move to the music, and not worry about steps or some old guy pushing them around. They enjoy themselves and sometimes take up the whole floor so there isn't hardly room for couple dancing. They don't really need me and that's fine if they're having fun.

Besides, many of these elderly ladies are too stove-up to move faster than a middle-aged sloth—which still isn't too shabby if a ninety-five-year-old gal can move as fast as any middle-aged creature. I might be a sloth some day, but I'm not now, so I'm open for a more lively scenario.

This exposure here at the old folks home reminded me of my dancing in the distant past and motivated me to think about expanding my dance experience. But if I don't know anything but the polka, where would I dance, who would I dance with, and how would I know what to do? Would dance lessons be the best option?

Chapter Four
Western Swing

The idea of lessons both excited and scared me. I knew I was absurdly tardy at age eighty-six in getting around to formal instruction. But my desire was growing stronger, and I figured that If I could ski from Idaho to Wyoming across the Teton Mountain Range in my seventies, I could learn how to boogie in my eighties. So I figured I was ready—or was I?

And this is when my telemarking ski buddy, Monte, came into the picture. We had done lots of crazy and fantastic ski outings, but I hadn't known he was also an inveterate dancer, having started way back in high school. When he found out I had a hankering to kick up my heels like he was doing, he made me an offer—that I *should have* refused. Monte is a true friend, but he had way too much confidence in my learning ability.

He took me to a series class of his Western Swing club. He explained that I would start in the third week of a four week group lesson, which meant that I would already be two weeks behind all the other students. *What was I thinking?!* That's like taking a freshman junior varsity football player from the bench and putting him in the second half of a varsity game.

Incredibly there was another first timer there, a woman, as clueless as I, who volunteered to partner with me. We floundered around, messed up the turns as we scrambled a step or two behind the rest of the class. After that initial fiasco I went downstairs to the main ballroom. To me it looked like hundreds of people and as far as I could tell, they all just came fresh from *Dancing With The Stars*. I was overwhelmed, frozen to my chair, too chicken to approach any of those dancing madonnas, so I prevailed upon poor Monte to put me out of my misery and get me home.

But Monte is a faithful friend and wants others to have as much fun as he does. And he doesn't give up easily. "Come with me next Sunday," he told me. "There are three nice lady friends I sit with. They are in their seventies and like to dance the slow ones. They would be glad to help you."

That sounded like more my speed, so I agreed to go. The ladies were really helpful and were willing to put up with my inexperience and give me pointers. We just did the basic *two step,* slow ones, and that's as far as I got. I watched a variety of dancers there doing turns and swing and a lot of neat-looking stuff. It was exciting and inspiring and I wanted to have as much fun as they were having. In my impatience I seemed to have forgotten that my dance level was a lowly *Klutz 1*.

I complained to Monte that I wanted to try something a little faster and more stimulating.

"Go ask Susie or Lucy to dance, they like to really hoof it up good," Monte advised. He was referring to a couple of younger women that he had introduced me to earlier.

I should mention here that besides being a *Klutz 1* dancer, I am also legally blind, so I protested. "I've just barely met them, and I'm not sure I could spot them," I said. "It's too hard for me to see which ones they are over there sitting with all those other people. I can't tell who they are until I get right in close, and I can't walk up and stick my face in front of every sweet young thing over there."

"Don't worry," Monte said, "I'll think of something."

Yeah, right, I thought. But a few minutes later Susie appeared in front of me."Would you like to dance?" she said sweetly. So I danced a faster two step, since that's all I knew. I braced myself and stuck my hand up and flung her out. Surprised, she nonetheless spun around gracefully with a giggle that expressed a reaction of *what the hell was that?!* —not even close to a response like *oh, great move!*

A few minutes later the other gal, Lucy, came over and invited me to dance. Appropriately humbled, I didn't try anything fancy. But still I wondered: What's the deal? Did Monte slip them a few bucks or what?

So I asked him. "I told them," Monte said, "that, with your poor vision, the only way you could find them was to come up and start feeling and touching them."

Wow, so that's what got them over here so fast. Hmm … I pondered. I then visualized a scenario: If I got up and walked towards all those ladies sitting over there, I bet I could make them scatter like a six year old running through a flock of chickens!

Chapter Five

Las Vegas To Polka

This time, Monte ventured a different offer. It was the *Las Vegas Polka Fest,* a huge national event offered only once a year. Monte is not a polka buff, but a friend had persuaded him to go, promising that they also did western swing as well as polka. I thought, *a Polka Fest, what's not to like about that!* Monte had already reserved a double room, so I tagged along.

As we entered the first ballroom where our assigned table was, I could feel the vibrant energy and collective passion for dancing. Even better, there seemed to be a variety of available women to dance with. One was called Lucy. I thought maybe she was older than she looked, because she was wearing pretty heavy makeup to disguise her middle aged complexion. Once after a western swing two step, she asked me, "Do you rock n' roll?" I wasn't sure what she meant. Maybe that was code for something kinky.

"Probably not," I answered evasively. Late in the evening on my way back to my hotel room I saw her with a guy, apparently on the way to his room, so I was glad I had previously answered her question negatively. The next day when I saw her in the ballroom, I asked, "Are you Juicy Lucy—or just Lucy?"

"Just … Lucy," she muttered. Then i regretted saying that to her. It was none of my business and I should never assume. Maybe Lucy wasn't Juicy, as I had speculated; perhaps she was like the majority of the folks there, just regular polka dancers having fun.

For, indeed, the polka dancing was fantastic, with hooting and hollering and an impressive variety of dancers, including some doing the distinctive *Dutch hop* that I had first seen years ago in Denver. I watched their technique, but could not do it myself when I tried to imitate that style of dancing.

A few times Monte and I left the dance venue and went to the *Strip* to take in a *Cirque du Soleil* show. We also went to other Vegas attractions that were free.

I thought the whole weekend was a hoot. But the following year when I asked Monte if he wanted to go to the Polka Fest, he answered, "No thanks. Too damn many polkas."

Monte is a *smooth dancer,* not a *hopping dancer.*

Back to Western Swing

After the Polk Fest I went to a few more western swing dances with Monte, but it became so obvious that his crowd were all long time dancers who were there to dance and socialize, not to teach beginners.

I told Monte that what I needed was—actual instruction. So persistent Monte talked Patricia, one of his dance friends, into coming over to his garage one day so they could give me a lesson on initiating a simple turn for the lady. They were patient, but we didn't have a lot of time and I couldn't seem to coordinate my feet and hands with my brain. It seemed obvious to me that if I really wanted to learn to dance well, I should commit myself to a series of lessons with a professional dance studio.

Chapter Six
Lies and Vacillations

After only six weeks of lessons I had mastered the rhumba, the cha cha, single time swing, triple time swing, hustle, Lindy hop, bachata and waltz.

And if you believe that, I have a great investment for you: Triple returns; all you have to do is slip two thousand bucks in cash to me today before midnight. Hurry so you won't miss this one chance in a million to become filthy rich and obnoxious.

Maybe if you were rehearsing for six weeks, day and night for a role in *Dirty Dancing* or *Saturday Night Live* you could learn that fast, But for the rest of us mortal earthlings it takes considerable time and dedication. Dancing is an art and requires practice, building one skill on top of another. Attaining those skills is a challenge, but it's also fun and gratifying. I knew all of this, and had no doubt that I should sign up for formal instruction.

But—when I contemplated the reality of dance lessons, I felt the anxiety creeping in, shoving aside my resolve. Where the hell was all that mountaineering bravado? Damn! I must have contracted fainthearted *flatlanditis* in this lower elevation!

That's why I equivocated and procrastinated. Besides starting dance lessons at my advanced age, there were other concerns which made me hesitate. One disadvantage I had was my short stature. Women like to be with men taller than they, especially when paired off on the dance floor

And do you know how many tall women are walking around here in this twenty-first century?! I'm fully convinced that at one point in our cosmos, God must have decreed that She wanted more tall women on Earth. I don't remember such a large gaggle of elongated girls when I was in high school. Most of them were appropriately petite, with just a few who were about eye to eye with me or taller.

Now stay with me, for this is relevant. Scientists know that all dinosaurs became extinct at the same time because an asteroid smashed into the earth. The proof was in the strata of rocks. Before the asteroid hit, the strata was full of dinosaur fossils. After the date of the asteroid collision there were none.

Geological strata can reveal much about all species. So I bet that if archeologists thousands or millions of years in the future were to compare the stratum of the year 1940 with the stratum of 2020 and afterward, they would see that the 2020 human female fossils were much longer. It's notable that the time span between those two dates is less than a blip in geologic time. But as they say, that old gal, you know, God, she works in mysterious ways.

However, I am grateful to our merciful Creatress that She didn't decree that all short girls become extinct. It just seems like it when us vertically challenged guys are looking for a complimentary dance partner.

The irony is that I come from a family of tall men. My grandfathers, my father, and my brother were all six footers. Even my sisters were not what you would call petite. I know I have tall genes within me, because I unselfishly passed them all to my three sons, who are five feet ten, to six feet one. And they didn't get it from their mother, who was short, like her parents.

So what happened to me? My mother was five feet tall and she passed her legs to me. Maybe she thought I was destined to become a personage of such importance that she wanted to keep me humble. My daughter is petite, but so beautiful that maybe mom wanted her to be humble too.

All well and good, but back to dancing now. A more mundane problem was my baggy pants. I don't have any hips to speak of so the pants slide down, and that can look a bit slovenly. I cinch my belt tightly, but with movement, down go my britches! And my butt isn't big enough to fill up the slack.

On a ski tour or hike it doesn't matter, but baggy pants on the dance floor beside an attractive, stylishly dressed woman with a nice derriere, the contrast must be distressing to look at.

However, I would soon learn that this oversized-pants issue was as inconsequential as a speck of mildew on the windowsill on a hot Sacramento summer morning. Until recently I didn't know about the stores that sell all sizes, including slim fit pants.

Another epiphany that reduced my anxiety occurred when I watched certain short guys dancing with taller women: If you are a really good dancer, it doesn't matter how short or how old you are—the ladies want you! —To dance with them. What a great motivation this is to work hard on my dancing!

I would also find out that there are gracious tall women who are perfectly willing to dance with us compact guys and even grace us with a welcoming smile on their friendly faces. People who enjoy dancing are usually nice folks, tall or short.

So I finally abandoned my faint hearted attitude. Baggy pants be damned! What the hell, if I learned the telemark jump turn in my sixties, I can learn how to dance in my eighties!

Guest Writers

Before I describe my belated but brave entry into the realm of ballroom dance, I would like to remind you that *everyone* has a story, each one unique to that individual, with varying perspectives. I talk to a lot of my fellow dancers, and some of them said it was okay to share their stories with you. I now invite you to enjoy the first one of these engaging tales about their dancing exploits. Haideh was the first to submit her story, so she has *first dibs,* and sets the tone nicely for the ones to follow.

Haideh's Story

I always loved dancing but didn't think I could dance well. I had tried ballroom dancing with my husband but he wasn't into it and after a few lessons, we stopped going.

Sometime after my husband died, I looked for dance venues close to me but was unable to find the right place. A year later, I went on a date with a fellow who treated me to a private dance lesson with a fine teacher. Though my date ended up not being the right fit, the dance teacher was a perfect match.

I first focused on salsa and practiced dancing weekly with a very friendly group in Placerville. Then I discovered east coast swing and focused more on swing and its varieties for another six to eight months, going to Midtown Barfly and occasionally to the Sacramento Ballroom.

I had heard from two sources about Arthur Murray, and on August 20, 2018, I went to Folsom and had a lesson with Wesley. It was a match made in heaven. I fell in love. Now multiply that by seven or more and that's how I felt after dancing with and learning from each of the other amazingly talented dance instructors, and the owner and coach at Arthur Murray in Folsom.

I should emphasize that this is by no means an attempt to advertise them and no one has asked me to promote Arthur Murray. A funny story on this: Just recently an online date asked me if I was really interested in him or if I was recruiting for my dance studio!

I love this location, the friendly atmosphere, management, all the instructors, teaching methods, activities, and, last but not least, the students who come here. It's a safe and loving environment. It feels like home and like family.

Learning to dance using the right form and proper technique is not only beautiful but also keeps the body parts moving comfortably.

Chapter Seven

Beginning Dance Lessons

Despite my dauntless determination, it was with more angst than valor the first time I, the past-his-prime octogenarian, walked into the Arthur Murray Folsom Dance Center for my trial lesson. But it went well and the teacher's skilled and calm geniality helped quell my nervousness.

But I was still lacking in confidence and patience. In one of my first full lessons I was trying to learn how to give the lady a simple, outside turn, and I kept messing it up. "That's okay," my teacher said.

"It's not okay," I retorted, "I want to do it right!"

"It's okay because you're learning," she said.

Yeah . . .good point. I shouldn't be so hard on myself. So I kept learning, but it would still be a long time before I would be up to the level of Patrick Swayze in *Dirty Dancing*. Maybe five lifetimes from now?

The common reaction I get when I tell someone I've started dancing is, "Oh, dance lessons, huh? That must be good exercise!"

Pshaw, I think, *not as much as I get at the gym.* It's the brain that gets the workout, and that is good. I can almost feel my brain whirring away like a washer on a spin cycle, trying to process all the information my instructors have thrown into it. *Okay,* my brain cries, *we got it up here and now I'm passing it along. Let's see if your body parts and muscles are as smart as I am.*

Research has shown that ballroom dancing can help prevent Alzheimer's disease. Dancing involves different brain functions at the same time: Each of these functions is handled differently by the brain, which helps develop different neural paths. Physical exercise can produce new brain neurons, but then the brain needs a challenge to use these new neurons.

I'm afraid that the grayer the hair of the learner, the harder his gray matter has to work. It is a real challenge for those brain cells who thought they'd earned the right to sit back and be lazy. But the brain is like any other working part: stop using it and it ceases to function properly.

The brain works in different ways for different people, so we don't all learn the same way. Some students can benefit from a verbal explanation. For example, here's how a teacher might explain to me a move called the *cross body lead:* "You're at a right angle with her, then you move sideways to the left while she moves forward. You see, you turn away from her, leading her to pass in front of you while dancing across from one side of your body to the other."

But here's what I thought I heard: *The Dynamics of a Spinning Top shows possible values of the angular momentum vector, in the non-inertial body frame, for a free, asymmetric top. The ellipsoid is … blah blah blah.*

And some people are good at learning from watching. When my teachers provide a demonstration for a new move, my reaction may be, *wow, that looked neat, but I have no idea what the hell they did.* Or I could think, *yeah, so cool and it doesn't look that hard either.* But when I try it, suddenly it's like trying to ski with one foot in a ski and the other in a snowshoe.

I've about decided that the only way I can learn is to kidnap a comely lass and make her dance the new move with me 262 times. Well, I would never really kidnap anyone, but the 262 times is about right.

Repetition is how I learned the telemark jump turn. But I didn't need a partner, so I went out onto the snow and did 1,234 jump turns. I think I fell about 803 times, but then I started to get it, and finally it was registered in my muscle memory.

Enough spiel about my skiing; let's hear now from skier/dancer, Kris.

Kris's Story

Dancing of some sort has threaded throughout my life. It was mostly rock and roll and slow dancing, like the waltz. This was without formal training, just moving to the beat of the music; that's what I love to do! Doesn't everyone? All kinds of music—except rap—not rap! Can anyone even dance to rap?

My earliest memories of dance were my parents' desire for me to be a ballerina. So with ballerina drawings all over my bedroom, it seemed I was predestined to do this form of dance.

When I went to the ballet studio, I was observing the graceful lines and movements of the teenage ballerinas, and managed to let my tiny fingers linger a bit too long in the door jamb, and as the door slammed on them I screamed like I was being tortured, and thereafter refused to ever return to such a place of pain.

After my mother's dream to make me into a ballerina was squelched, she sent me to the Byron Ryder School of Dance, a ballroom class for preteens, and that was more to my liking. The room was large and grand, the music was soft and lyrical (classical?), and Mr. Ryder was tall, thin and firm, as he guided his young students around the floor. What a good leader he was! It was amazing how he swept me around that ballroom; it was so easy to . . . just follow— truly magical!

Yes, a great dancer but an unkind man. I left after he repeatedly berated the other students who happened to be less athletic than me.

After this early introduction, I went to the more current trends for modern music. Nothing technical or formal—just rocking to the music of the day.

There was one other tidbit of dance that I was privy to watch and do. My grandparents enjoyed doing the polka. While in their teens, each left the folk dances of the old country and came across the ocean to embrace the polka dancing popular in America. They were good dancers and fun to watch. I learned from them and other family members at weddings and other family events. A polka band was often close by and that beat sends my feet a-flying still today.

Currently, my newest dance experience is with Arthur Murray. I have been introduced to many new-to-me ballroom dances. The Latin dances have a wonderful beat and I never knew there were so many variations. The more mainstream dance types like tango, foxtrot and waltz are really fun too. And of course the *swing* that I just see as good ol' rock n' roll. My favorite of these dances is the one I am doing at any moment in time. I cannot say there is an overall favorite. It is all just the aerobic joy of moving to the beat of the music.

Chapter Eight
The Search for A Practice Partner

I can learn a skiing move alone, but I can't practice a dance move without a partner. Sure I can work on a few specific steps by myself, but this is couples dancing, not single freestyle, break dancing, or vodka-induced fantasy dancing.

So . . . the logical solution, it seemed to me, was to go find a practice partner. Yeah, sure, but where? I'm not going to the mall or a bar and walk up to a woman I've never met and ask, "Hey would you like to come with me and practice dancing?" No, these days there are apps and websites and other electronic monstrosities for practically everything. In this case it was called *Dancepartners.com*. I enrolled and thus my naive and impatient nature brought me to an arena full of social landmines.

How many sprightly ladies do you think are looking for a half blind, eighty-six year old novice dancer who can't even drive to the dance hall?

Right. So I had to cheat . . . just a little: In my profile, I lied about my age, saying I was in my seventies. Not too far fetched, as many people have guessed me to be about that age. But I did admit the non-driving part.

I got responses from three nice ladies over the course of a few months. My strategy was to invite them to lunch at my senior community to get acquainted. After talking with me and seeing that I was not a shambling old derelict, they would then hear my confession about my real age, and that seemed to work out okay.

I took the first lady to a big Arthur Murray dance in a hotel that cost me some big bucks for the two of us, which was ridiculously expensive for a so-called first date. Then when we danced she was not only underwhelmed by my dancing prowess, but also admitted that all the driving it would take to cart me around would be too much.

The second lady was attractive and affable, but having to chauffeur me from one dance venue to another was a deal breaker, since she resided some distance away.

The third woman, Jacquline, was younger, lived a lot closer, was willing to drive. and didn't care how *mature* I was, as long as she "had somebody to go to dances with."

This scheme of mine for partner matching was as brilliant an idea as inviting my friends to a beach party in Nova Scotia, Canada, on New Year's Eve. The flaw in my strategy was the fact that all these ladies, including Jaqueline, had much more dancing experience than I. I'm supposed to be the leader, so it was all backwards, kind of like a sixth grader learning arithmetic trying to teach his math teacher algebra.

Predictably, at our first trial dance together, my new partner started correcting me. "You're not doing that rhumba step right . . . no, that's not when I do the turn." She was trying to help me, but with her talking, my concentration was shot and any confidence I had stored up dissipated like confetti in a Santa Ana wind.

A few days later she suggested that we go to the Sunday night Elks Club dance that started at six and lasted until midnight. "There will be a lot of dancers there," she said excitedly, "and I want to help you and all, but I also want to dance a lot with *advanced* dancers."

Instinctively I balked. *Six to twelve? Sunday night? That's the night my son comes over, and besides, that's way too long and way too late.*

How was I going to escape from this self-made predicament without shattering her hopes? I've heard there are *"Fifty ways to leave a lover,"* but I wasn't a lover, and wasn't about to *slip out the back, Jacquline.* She had been so enthusiastic to have a partner and so willing to come pick me up, and after only a couple of weeks here I am abandoning this whole project that I had worked so hard to achieve.

But when I gently announced my desire to terminate our partnership, she took it well. I mean *really* well . . . her body language said, "Oh, *thank God!*" So we parted amicably.

Now let's move on to another story; this time from Yuriko and her first exposure to dance.

Yuriko's Story

Growing up in Japan, my earliest exposure to dancing was a tradition called *Bon Odori*, which takes place all over Japan every summer. Originally a religious ceremony to honor one's ancestors, in modern times that aspect is nearly forgotten amidst such joyous dancing and jubilant celebration. Whole communities take part, and families with children and grandparents gather in the town square or temple, wearing a traditional cotton Kimono called *Yukata*. The dances are easy to learn, so everyone, men, women, and children do the *Bon Odori*.

Sometimes more experienced dancers are on a platform with lanterns all around, and the rest of the folks dance in a circle around it. People come together not only to dance but also to enjoy the evening visiting with each other.

Many years later, now residing in the U.S., I had the opportunity to dance again. My neighbor's daughter, an experienced ballroom dancer, took me to a dance party at a ballroom studio. I was asked to dance by a very accomplished dancer, and despite my limited ballroom experience, I was astonished to realize that I was actually dancing—spinning, twirling, and even shimmying. All that good stuff I didn't even know I could do. I learned that night that a good leader can make you look good, even when you're doing moves you didn't know.

I used to think that once you learned to dance, that was it. But then I realized that there are many levels of dancing and that there is no end—it's unlimited. But that's okay, because there's joy at every level and you can make progress all your life.

Another surprise I had was that dance moves are not preplanned—it's up to the leader, his responsibility and his choice. And you are the follower, so you have to—yes, follow. That doesn't fit my personality, so it's difficult. I have to wait to see what he's going to do next. And definitely don't try to lead the leader or your invitations to dance may dry up.

Although dancing etiquette isn't always observed by everyone at our practice parties, I find it very nice. I still remember one young man, still in high school, would do it with great finesse. Looking you straight in the eye, and with a perfect stance, he would extend his hand as the invitation to dance with him. After the dance he would take your hand in his arm, return you to your seat, and thank you. And of course, he was a great dancer. Wouldn't it be nice if this kind of graceful courtesy was commonplace!

Dancing is challenging, physically and mentally. It requires concentration, coordination, balance and agility. It keeps your mind and body active and engaged. It offers so many benefits.

It's also fun, and makes you smile, makes you laugh, makes you appreciate music, makes you stand up straight, lifts your spirits, and gives you confidence.

Our fellow dancers and teachers at my studio are so encouraging and appreciative of our efforts. They always praise us profusely for our performance no matter how it turns out. They're the best cheer leaders ever. They are the most crazy, uninhibited, fun-loving extroverts. To me, that is the best part.

Chapter Nine
Back to The Basics

If our American culture favored dancing from an early age, like in Japan, maybe I could have avoided my failed fantasy to prematurely find that perfect dance partner. I had not left Arthur Murray but my search had distracted me. Now I was ready to concentrate on my lessons, resolved to work and play hard to become a dancer. It would be strictly ballroom from now on, with lessons, and serious learning and blood letting.

As the lessons progressed, I became aware of another of my deficiencies, which could be described as *musculoskeletal distortion* in the neck, and lower and upper back. Put simply it just means *poor posture*. Many of us experience this condition, especially as we get older. Our back curves, our head drops down and we hunch our shoulders. It may happen slowly over the years without our giving it a thought. During this gradual remolding of our body, it starts out like a young plant that is proud and straight. But when a cornstalk doesn't get enough water it starts to wilt, bend and shrink. This is what happens to us as we age. But if we impose a little irrigation in the form of exercise, stretching and a daily consciousness of holding ourselves more erect, we can mitigate this aging process.

I used to tell people that I don't need to drink much water because I'm a camel and I store it in the hump on my back. (They don't really, it's fat.) Whether that was ever a clever remark is doubtful, but for sure now it no longer strikes my funny bone.

Most of the old folks in my senior community are at least a little bent over, and some a *lot*. But you can also see younger people with this slump hump. If you hunch over habitually, the fascia remolds itself in that position. Then you may not be able to straighten up even if you try.

Like when your dear mother use to say,"Don't make nasty faces, because if you keep doing it, it'll stay that way!"

I have to remember to correct my posture repeatedly every day, because after several decades of slumping, good posture feels unnatural. Except for disease, slumping for most people is principally habit.

Therefore my dance instructors have to keep after me. "Do that move again but stand up straight." It got to be such a constant reminder that now all they have to do is an upward hand signal. They also impressed on me the fact that when my head is up, I'm "two inches taller." That's a great motivation for a *heads-up!*

Instructor Gerard gave me the best description for good posture when he said, to "keep your head over your heart." When you do this, your position achieves a three pronged posture correction: your chin is tucked, your head is up and your back is straight.

There is nothing more revealing than to watch a video of yourself dancing. As I was doing a certain routine, I thought I was moving well. But when I viewed the video, I saw an old man doing a polka. Yes, I know, I *am* an old man, but that doesn't mean I have to move like a decrepit old dog at the end of his days. I live an active life, and I don't have to carry myself like I'm one hundred and twenty years old. It's just habit!

How could I have improved this routine? I was able to pinpoint two actions that were correctable: keep my body erect with my head up, chin tucked a little, and stay light on the balls of my feet, rather than flat footed on my heels. If I could do the same routine again with those changes, the video would show an instant rejuvenation!

Role Reversal

This is an interesting switch. I spent thirty-one years teaching young people. Now young people are teaching me. Shortly before I retired these young ladies were infants or possibly no more than an eager smile on their parents' faces. Now they have me, a great- grandfather, as their dance student.

But I am not complaining. On the contrary, I feel fortunate. My instructors are competent, caring, professional, affable and patient. After working with them for several weeks they also seem like friends. The positive environment of the dance studio is uplifting and it's fun to mix with the other students, all younger than me. This helps to keep me young. Groucho Marx once said, "You're only as old as the girl you feel." What I say is, "I'm only as old as the girl I'm dancing with."

In the next story, I think most of us can relate to Ruxandra's insecurities about starting a new, and unexplored activity.

Ruxandra's Story

Being in front of people terrifies me. So, when my friend asked me to accompany her to a group dance class my first instinct was to tell her "No." The problem was I was in the middle of a very messy breakup with my ex and all I had been doing for weeks was sitting in my half-put-together apartment moping about what to do with my time. So, I told her "Ok."

For days leading up to the open house I kept coming up with reasons for why I shouldn't go. I had too much work. I didn't know anyone else there. What if I messed something up and people laughed at me? That was really my biggest fear.

The day of the dance, I agonized over what to wear. What if I didn't fit in with everyone? Did I have the right shoes? What sort of shoes does one even wear to dance? Should I wear pants? A skirt? What do I even do with my hair?

I showed up to the class a full forty-five minutes early and sat in the parking lot in my car watching people go inside. Twenty minutes before the class I went in and sat nervously on a bench against a wall, palms sweating and trying to avoid too much eye contact, lest someone should talk to me.

That was short lived. Immediately, one of the instructors greeted me brightly and started to engage in conversation. I felt at ease as more people arrived and I eventually met up with my friend. I felt safe with her around and when the group class started, I found myself laughing and having a good time.

The practice party was an entirely new experience and a new wave of panic washed over me. I didn't know any of these other dances that were being announced. I was resigned to turn into a wall flower, but that also was not meant to be. Students and instructors asked me to dance, regardless of whether I knew the steps or not and by the end, when one of the instructors asked me to come to a free lesson, I instantly said "Yes."

And that was the beginning of a very strange journey where I would push my comfort zone a little farther every day; learn how to be more comfortable in my own skin; and meet some truly incredible people that I never expected to touch my life in such a meaningful way.

Chapter Ten

Private Lessons

    I think many of us are unsure of ourselves when we are about to jump into a new episode of our lives. Getting out on that dance floor for the first time can be nerve-wracking. That's why private lessons are valuable. You're working one on one, can ask all the questions you want and make mistakes that nobody else sees. Repetition is part of the learning process, so you can repeat the move as many times as you need to.

    My instructors at Arthur Murray do not criticize, but they do correct: "Let's try that again. Remember, the left foot forward, then cha cha cha, then the right foot back."

    When you're learning, you're going to screw up sometimes, if you're human. When you do, don't beat yourself up about it—(like I do). Those flubs can actually be a source of humor—even if it's after the fact. My teachers are always encouraging, whether I'm dancing like a star or messing it up like a dweeb.

If you have a spouse or a partner who is willing to have lessons together, it's nice because besides splitting the cost of the lesson, the two of you can practice the new moves after the lesson.

One night I was having a joint lesson in the w*est* coast swing. In this dance style the leader has his right hand up, palm forward, to give his partner a *sugar push* on her left palm. But man, I didn't realize how dangerous some moves could be! My instructor cautioned me that I'd better "lower that hand a bit" when I'm doing the *sugar push* because I had it at chest level. "If your hand slipped it might end up where you don't intend."

No, don't want that! So I lowered my hand.

"Not that much lower," she said, "that could be even worse!!

(Outta the fryin' pan and into the fire!)

On another occasion, I nearly got myself into an even worse jam with some potentially dire consequences. It was a brand new move for me, called the *figure eight.* I was supposed to stay in place keeping my hand on my partner's back, while she was turning back and forth. But I moved and my hand erred involuntarily to her . . . front.

"Oh, no, Harvey," Brandi laughed, "you do that again and you'll have to ask her to go steady, maybe even give her a ring!"

But I seem to have escaped the aforementioned dire consequences. The lady still talks to me and has made no demands.

My mind—or maybe my body (maybe both)—works in mysterious ways sometimes that I don't understand. We were practicing the *country two step,* which is *slow-slow-fast-fast.* suddenly, Brandi said, "Harvey, when did you start walking like John wayne?"

"Huh?"

"Your slow steps are way too big."

"Oh, I wasn't aware of that."

"Don't worry, you'll correct it easily and it will be perfect."

"That'l be the day," I said in my best attempt to imitate*The Duke.*

The Wayward Thumb

Another tip for my fellow leaders: *Keep that thumb under control*. It wants to grab. It doesn't mean to, but we guys are used to getting a good grasp on things. We grab the hammer to pound, we get a good grip on the baseball bat to score a homer. We are used to relying on our handy thumbs, but now they tell us its use is forbidden!

Our thumb is called *opposable* because it can be moved around to touch the other fingers, and that's what gives us the ability to . . . *grasp*. You may clasp your honey's hand tightly and lead her through the garden path to the park bench. Yes, this special digit is so important that it differentiates us primates from all other species.

But if you grab your dancing partner with it while doing a maneuver it will be uncomfortable and may even twist the nice lady's wrist. Besides, it limits the action you're trying to perform and might make it look awkward.

You want smooth transitions with just your palm or fingers that slide neatly across her hand as it pivots with easy fluency to get to the desired position.

If it's a complete turn you may even use the *cup and pin* technique with her hand being the cup and two of your fingers being the pin as one of you spins around. Easy does it; remember, this is not jiu jitsu. It's dancing.

I can write about this, but that doesn't mean I'm always faithful in observing it. So, gentlemen, if you fail to heed this above admonishment, I advise you to keep an eye on your dance instructor. I speak from experience. It's likely that she is holding a roll of tape as a first warning. If you ignore that, she's liable to tape that misbehaving maverick in place; and if you think your thumb resents a simple scolding, how much will he like to be hogtied?

When my opposable digit forgets his proper role and starts to clutch instead of hide, I see my dedicated teacher—twirling a big roll of blue tape, plastic, very sturdy looking—twirling, twirling. That's all it takes. She wins: Instructor 1, thumb 0. That is, until the next time.

Now let's   check out a married couple's foray into the ballroom scene. Maybe they got a bit of a late start, but they made up for that and are still going strong.

Stan And Lynn's Story

"Line up everyone, it's time for the foxtrot mixer!" These are words designed to terrify. While we weren't exactly dance-phobic, we had a healthy respect for the dance floor; healthy respect meaning that we never ventured out there. If we went someplace where dancing was happening, we would just sit quietly and watch.

Our first brush with Arthur Murray came when our oldest son got engaged. He and his fiancée arrived at our house one Saturday afternoon bubbling with enthusiasm from their first lesson in the foxtrot. They joyfully showed us the magic left turn there in our family room. We quickly decided to get ourselves over to Arthur Murray as well, especially as Stan might be expected to dance with the bride. So we signed up for our first slate of lessons, which came with Monday night parties and Friday night parties. Still not sure of ourselves, we hated the foxtrot mixers. As these things often go, our son and his fiancée broke up. But we kept up with our lessons for another year and learned enough to not have to always sit on the sidelines.

When we retired from teaching and started going on cruises, we saw there is always dancing. We wanted to be able to do more than the few basic steps we knew, so we called Arthur Murray Folsom.

We immediately realized how much we had forgotten and how much we wanted to know. The studio was full of enthusiastic young teachers who were willing to help a couple of old folks. Since then it has filled our lives, getting us out and getting us moving two or three times a week. We've had several instructors, and they each have contributed something important to our dancing. Now we are unafraid of dance floors and often get compliments on cruises. As for the terrifying foxtrot mixers, that's in the past too.

Chapter Eleven
The Frankenstein Boot

If Stan and Lynn didn't like the fox trot mixer at first, I wonder how they would like doing that caper in a huge, long, heavy stiff blasphemy-engendering boot. I could tell them.

What an unwelcome interruption that was! My dancing had ben no longer jinxed— I was beginning to shake out the kinks. It was springtime and the grass was greening, the trees were budding, bees were buzzing and I was breaking into song— which was cut short by a piteous pain from my achilles tendon. It was begging me to stop the fancy footwork at dances, and stay off the StairMaster at the gym.

And thereby began my bout with the abominable boot. "How long?" I asked the podiatrist.

"As long as six months'" he said, as though he were a dentist simply telling me to wait a couple of hours for the numbness wore off before chewing.

Six months, are you insane? HE wasn't but I would be. No dancing, no walking to the gym for workouts? They call this grotesque stomp-master a *walking boot*. You can walk to the bathroom, or to the dining room, but not a mile to the gym or execute a back rock in an east coast swing; and forget the polka! What am I going to do?! Ah, then I remembered good old FART, (Folsom Area Rapid Transit). It would at least get me to the gym for some modified workouts. Heck of a lot better than sitting in my recliner as my body parts atrophy.

But I was still missing my dance lessons, so, suffering the symptoms of withdrawal after a month, I stomped into the dance center one day, begging for a fix. I looked so pathetic they couldn't turn me down.

In my imagination during this lull, I had convinced myself that I was better than I really was, and didn't want to forget all those smooth moves. But *smooth* would be a lousy description for my movements while wearing the boot. It was the opposite of *trip the light fantastic*. Well, maybe the word *trip* would be appropriate. When I lifted that left leg, it felt like there was six pack of Budweiser attached to the boot that was holding my leg captive. A simple *back rock* with that foot was impossible. Oh well, the lesson was worthwhile to hold on to some muscle memory.

But the regrettable result of the tendon treatment was that after two and a half months wearing the *Unbearable Boot,* the tendon was no better, but my arthritic back started whining, *What the hell are you doing to me?* And my left heel, heretofore healthy, got as sore as a bad toothache. So on a Wednesday in July I shucked the Monster and on Saturday I went to the mountains and did some short hikes with family. I felt a little discomfort, but no severe pain. Soon the back and heel pains disappeared. Ever since then, including at the time of this writing, I have been stretching the tendon and calf daily and have gained my little world back.

Once more at my regular dance lessons I resumed my practice of entertaining my instructors with my maverick missteps and miscues.

Even though my achilles tendon still has not completely healed, the pain is so slight that I am rarely aware of it while dancing or during my gym workouts, and not even when I dance the polka. That's why I was surprised one day during a lesson when my teacher asked me if my ankle hurt. "No" I said,. "It's okay."

"Oh . . . I thought you were . . . limping a little."

Although she didn't say so, I can only assume that my dancing that day must have looked especially lame.

But I was not discouraged. My teachers are marvelous and for an old dude with no real dance skills when I started (except for polka), I was learning more than I thought possible.

And now Gail will regale us with an account about a remarkable resumption of her dance life.

Gail's Story

Many years ago I took jazz, tap and ballet lessons, did performances, got married —and stopped dancing for twenty-six years. Then, there I was, a divorcee, on my own, and thought, *why not start dancing again?*

There were no evening classes available in those dances I had done, but on the way home from work, a building with *Arthur Murray Dance Center* caught my eye. But I didn't know much about ballroom, and there are always more women than men; and I didn't know how I'd feel about dancing with women.

Finally, two years later, November of 2017, with encouragement from someone special, I walked into the studio on the way home from work and was delighted that they offered 9 o'clock ballroom classes. The lady I talked to, who I later discovered was Kate, the studio owner, was very personable and encouraging, so I signed up for some introductory classes.

Later I joined a Merengue Formation, which was a choreographed class that met once a week. It was fun and I met more people. Brandi was the instructor, and, what a spunky and fun gal she was, as well as a great teacher! Brandi mentioned one day that I would need a black blouse with rhinestones, a black skirt, and silver, sparkly shoes.

What for?

We would be performing at the Holiday Extravaganza party the following month, so I was committed and just hoped for the best. It turned out to be great. I met some wonderful ladies, and never looked back. I had been bitten by the *dance bug.*

Some time later, Brandi introduced me to Harvey, another student, and we danced. *Poor Harvey,* I thought. I didn't know many dance moves and he was a good dancer. But he was encouraging with his brilliant smile, and he has become a lovely friend. We even take dance lessons together once a week, which is an enjoyable way to learn more moves and get more practice.

A month after the Extravaganza Party, my teacher left, so Brandi became my instructor, which was exciting. I learned waltz, tango, fox trot, hustle, rumba, country western, and a few others. I also learned an Argentine Tango dance routine that Brandi choreographed and performed with me. I still have fond memories of that routine—just one of many thrills along my journey.

Two months later I was about to go to a district *showcase* that Brandi had told me about. It would be in San Jose, attended by dancers from fifteen Northern California studios. It would include two days of dancing, judges' feedback, cocktails, posh dinners, and a pro show. Would all those people be friendly or snub the new dancers? Was my dancing good enough?

Well, I went. I danced ninety plus dances, many with mistakes and people bumping into me, which ruined my concentration. I had second thoughts about being here.

But as I danced more, I got more comfortable, did better and had a blast. Other dancers and instructors were surprisingly friendly and encouraging. After all, they were there with the same passion for dancing, and the energy in that ballroom was electrifying. I left feeling that it was *an experience of a lifetime.*

I went to more showcases, including one in London, with Harvey and two other students. There we went to the renowned Royal Albert hall to watch the international Latin dance championships, and even got to dance on that famous ballroom floor. Another day Harvey and I dance the polka on the Westminster Bridge over the River Thames to bagpipe music.

In Seattle I danced my first competition, an event know as the *Dance-O-Rama.* Traveling around the world is just one of the perks of being in an Arthur Murray group. I have learned to have fun and not worry so much about mistakes. Our instructors don't criticize us for making mistakes so neither should we berate ourselves. Everybody messes up sometime.

Dancing with females isn't all that weird. In fact, some women are better leaders than some of the men. But the main thing is to keep smiling, which has been my motto for many years.

What a thrilling experience dancing continues to be! I have made friends, and found a community, much joy, and a passion!

Chapter Twelve
Group Classes

At first I thought the private lessons were a bit pricey until I found out that the lesson entitles you to attend a huge variety of group classes, offered five evenings a week, as well as the twice weekly evening *Practice Dances* and a Saturday afternoon dance.

Here's what to expect in a group class: "Leaders on this side and followers on the other side. Leaders always start on their left foot. Now, ladies, you always start on you right foot. Why? Because you're always—RIGHT!"

I think saying they're right gives the ladies an equality that perhaps they had not felt being the eternal *followers.*

Next the teacher shows the leaders the move, then repeats it as the leaders practice it. Then the followers learn their parts, and then you hear, "Okay, now go find a human," and the women come across to dance with the guys across from them.

After each trial, the ladies are told to "rotate" and move one notch to a different partner. This way you get to dance with a lot of different people, including the spouses who haven't chosen the option of staying with their hubby or wife. Most couples choose to rotate, and it's a good way to get better acquainted as well as experience a variety of leader styles.

Bless the newbies, for we all were there once. It can be especially intimidating for the guys.

"I'm not a leader," he says. "This is my first time." You practically have to pry him away from his safe place beside his wife standing on the followers side. He doesn't get it—that leader means —man or male. Face it, guys, it's our dance destiny, like it or not, to lead. And yeah, it seems like we have to learn the moves better than our female partners because we have to lead then into the correct pattern.

"How do you do this without feeling like a stick?" another guy asks. The answer probably is—you just keep doing it until it feels more human.

I sometimes wonder if I am afflicted with a *group-class-learning disability,* as I am probably one of the worst students in group. Even in skiing, my best outdoor sport in which I eventually excelled, my skill regressed when in a group telemark class. For some reason, that is just not the way I learn. I'm slow to catch on to a new move. Even if my brain gets it, my body parts and muscles don't cooperate quickly.

Also, I have trouble hearing and seeing, especially in a big class. Even now I sometimes opt for the smaller basic class to avoid getting so stressed.

My consternation was slightly placated one day when I overheard one of our senior instructors, a most experienced and a superb dancer, admit that he was always slower than others to catch on to a new move.

Still, it's embarrassing when we're being taught a routine and my partner and I end up facing east when all the others are facing west.

And then there are those things they call *head loops.* Those are strictly hand styling. The instructor demonstrated, and I could make out that his hands were flying around the woman's head and shoulders, but I couldn't tell what the heck he was doing. In the trial with a partner, I thought my hand was supposed to go on top of the woman's head. But the hand flap was supposed to be on her shoulder. Some women don't like you to touch their hair because it messes up their *do.* The instructor gently admonished me, saying "Oh, no Harvey, not on her head, that just looks like you're patting a child on her head, like "you're a nice little girl."

What the hell, they're called *head* loops, aren't they? But I call them *fruit loops,* because I don't like them.

Before each practice dance there is an *intermediate* and a *basic* group class. I stayed in the b*a*sic class for almost a year while I was learning. But the women gravitate to the *intermediate* after only a few lessons. I'll see a woman who was in the basic class one week as a beginner, and the following week, there she is, in the *intermediate,* just so perky and proud of herself! But the thing is, they can rely on the men to lead them, so that's easier.

But I also have to consider the possibility that females do a better job of picking up the footwork, rhythm, and poise quicker than the male gender.

But we all have our individual aptitudes, and us guys can excel in different ways. For example, men, especially after a couple of coffees or beers, do a better job of putting out the campfire when there's no other source of water available.

Guys Dancing with Guys

First of all, there is nothing kinky or unusual about this at a dance center. It's just that sometimes in a group class there are more males than females. That means that every few rotations some guy doesn't have a partner. If the instructor is female, she'll fill in for the missing partner so the guy doesn't have to go through the motions by himself. And . . . if the instructor is male, he can take the place of the missing partner in the same way. All the instructors, regardless of gender have to learn the parts of both leader and follower.

We manly guys often see women dancing with women, and don't think much about it. "Well, that's just what women do," we say. Who can understand women anyway?

But when there are two or more guys who are left without a partner at a practice party, do we dance with each other? Never. We are on the dance floor looking for a partner, here comes another guy. We quickly pass each other by, not even speaking. But it's not just a macho thing; we can't follow, so it wouldn't work anyway.

So, one night in a group class when there was a woman shortage and when they rotated I was isolated, womanless—partnerless. I hate that. The male instructor stepped in front of me to be my partner. At that time, the idea of my dancing with another guy was a concept I hadn't ever considered: I admit that initially I felt a little uncomfortable. But no one in the class took any notice of it, like it was no big deal, so I relaxed. The teacher rotated so he also partnered with other guys who were left without a female.

Another night, the lesson in this group class was the fox trot, and there were so few females in the small class that I was dancing with the male instructor every other rotation. He was encouraging and I felt comfortable.

Later in the evening at the practice party, they played a fox trot, but all the available women were dancing so I took a seat. The same male instructor from the group class came over and offered his hand. *Oh well, what the hell,* I thought, *why not?*

So I danced a whole dance with him. *Damn,* I thought, *this tall dude is really good! What a great follower!* The dance went well and he congratulated me at the end of it.

But, of course, it you asked me my preference, I'd still opt for one of these charming, young sixty-year-old lasses we have around here.

Next, you should be able to feel Tresa's passion and enthusiasm jumping out from the page.

Teresa's Story

I have loved dancing for years. I began college in 1977, studying dance. I thought I wanted to perform dance, however this wasn't meant to be. But still, if music is playing that has a catchy beat, I'm dancing, I'm moving!.

Two years ago I had a coupon for the Arthur Murray studio, and that's what first got me in the door. I had tried ballroom dance years before but didn't enjoy it that much. But that is not my opinion any longer! I have been blessed beyond measure since coming to Arthur Murray. I have returned to dance and LOVE LOVE LOVE it!!! I'm not performing but I am learning dance moves. Dancing makes me smile! Endlessly!

I get exercise with both body and mind. I have met great friends. I have challenged myself with skills that excite me. But most loved is having the friends!! We have found ourselves wanting more time together so we ride bikes, travel, bowl, camp, and do many other things together that keep driving our friendships even deeper.

Coming to Arthur Murray has changed my life and I just love it!!!

Chapter Thirteen
Practice Parties

Practice is what you need and practice is what you can get with a variety of partners at practice parties. Arthur Murray Folsom schedules practice parties on Wednesday and Friday nights, and Saturday afternoons. In general, the afternoon dances are less crowded and more casual.

But any of the practice parties give you a chance to hone your dancing skills. And if you have that uncommon skill of carrying on an intelligent dialog while executing a complex dance pattern, you can unload those clever gems of conversation you've been saving.

But if you're a leader and, like me, not good at multi-tasking, you may have to limit your scintillating conversation to break times or before and after the party.

"How are you tonight?" she asks. "Uh, fine, thanks."

"Did you have a nice thanksgiving?"

"Yes, we had it in San Rafael and the whole family was there."

Oh, damn, I got completely out of step then. I'd love to chat with this nice lady, but I have to figure out which move to do next. And I have to remember to stand tall, keep a good frame, not use my thumb, and avoid colliding with other couples. And you expect me to articulate an intelligent conversation ,too? Sure, you gals don't have to worry, all you have to do is relax, follow my lead and let me do all the thinking!

Sometimes if a partner wants to talk I just keep repeating the basic step and don't worry about the moves. That way I can enjoy talking with her, and get better acquainted, and that is perfectly fine. Can't do it every time though if I'm going to learn those dance patterns.

Beginning students may feel a bit intimidated at practice parties because they don't know all the dance styles yet. I would suggest they come anyway because the staff encourages the advanced students to help them and the instructors themselves are looking out for these self-conscious neophytes. I remember the days when I felt this insecurity:

"Why aren't you dancing this tango, Harvey?"

"All I know is the basic step."

"Then let's do just that. If you can spell you can dance the tango. Here we go. T-A-N—G-O! "Slow, slow, slow— quick, quick!"

Tango

We must remember to respect the mood of the tango. This is not a time for uncalled-for levity. (Or at least, don't make your jocularity too obvious.)

The tango is a distinctive dance style. The music is dramatic, captivating, serious and . . . sensual. The tango originated in lower-class districts of Buenos Aires, Argentina and Montevideo, Uruguay, and was frequently practiced in the brothels, then spread to the rest of the world.

The purists insist that when dancing the tango there should be *constant connection* through the body. The American Ballroom tango's frame is flexible, with not only the *close embrace* but also an open position. This open frame, similar to other dance styles, is what we're used to at Arthur Murray, since the closed position is too intimate to have with casual acquaintances or other people's spouses.

The *close embrace* involves intimate contact in the pelvis or upper thighs, but not the upper body. Followers are instructed to thrust their hips forward.

So this would be an appropriate setting in which to recount my tango experience one night with a lady who evidently was a *purist*— a follower of the intimate *closed embrace.*

I knew her name and that was all. She was possibly in her forties, blond, natural or bottle blond, how can you ever know for sure? She was a big boned lady, not fat, but substantial and taller than I, not someone I would want to get into a wrestling match with.

I was leading her in the open position and starting to execute a medio corte but she said, "You know, in the tango we have to be really close to do it well. Then she thrust her thigh between my legs. "There, you see? We have such good contact that I can tell with any movement where you're going with that move."

After my initial shock, I was mainly just a bit uncomfortable. "Yeah. okay," I stammered, "Well . . . I guess I don't mind if you don't." And so there we were, dancing, pelvis to pelvis as though we did it all the time. I don't remember any glorious or brilliant tango maneuvers; I think I was just a bit discomfited.

I don't believe she was trying to be sexy or provocative or intimate, I think she was sincere and out for a good time, doing the tango *the way* she thought *it should be done.*

I only saw her one time after that. It was the following week at another practice party. She went waltzing gayly by and threw out a cheery, "Hi Harvey," to me standing on the side. I thought, "Hello, tango tigress," but all I came up with was, "Oh…hi."

If you dance the tango, you know the move called *tango rock*. But did you know there is another species of this genre?

TANGO ROCK: An ancient stone artifact discovered in a remote mountainous area of Argentina.

This next dynamic couple advanced quickly, even to the point of competition.

Joel And Tierney's Story

After talking about taking dance lessons for years, Joel and I finally took our first lesson six months before our thirtieth wedding anniversary. Our first lesson was in December, 2017, and after the holidays we decided to take regular lessons. We were so bad we realized it would take awhile to feel competent.

Next thing we knew, we had to decide what path we wanted to take and what our goals were with Arthur Murray. We had no idea what a cha cha or a foxtrot was, nor most of the other dances for that matter. We enjoyed our lessons together, but it took time to figure out what the different dances were, what music went with the dance, and to remember what steps went where.

We attended group classes, which were uncomfortable at first. Practice dance parties for the first several months were a fiasco. We couldn't dance well enough to survive the songs, let alone enjoy ourselves for the entire forty-five minutes. We would try to figure out what we were supposed to do in a roomful of people, and many onlookers thought we were always fighting.

As former athletes, we both understood that just like anything, there is a large learning curve. Learning to dance together can be difficult, but dancing is a great new way to stay connected and do something active together that can last a lifetime. We loved being able to dance to our wedding song at our son's wedding in June, 2018, one day before our thirty-fifth anniversary, surrounded by family and friends. We have attended Arthur Murray events at the studio in Folsom, as well as events in Sacramento, San Jose, and Mexico. At our first *big* event in Sacramento, Joel got frustrated and walked off the dance floor while we were dancing the foxtrot. Our instructor came over and said, "You can't do that." Joel's response was, "We just did." Now we can laugh about that, and love having a wonderful, endorphin releasing, healthy hobby to do together.

Joel and I have made new friends, have learned how to dance rhythm and smooth dances, and have added a new dimension to our lives. We can let go of a taxing or emotional day and enjoy ourselves while we dance.

Taking lessons and going to events is expensive, but definitely worth the effort and sacrifice to keep music and dancing in our lives.

Chapter Fourteen
Graduation!

Arthur Murray has what they call *Medal* ratings. Each category, Bronze, Silver, and Gold, is made up of four levels. If I were ever to get as far as Bronze 3, I figure I would be a pretty good dancer. Can you imagine how good a Gold dancer must be?

So now it was time for my—graduation! But don't assume I was graduating from the tango! Maybe I wasn't a complete *tango virgin*, but I still had a long ways to go in tango as well as all the other dance styles. This graduation exercise was only on basic steps of three styles I had been working on.

So I assure you that this was far from being the apex of my dancing career. It was more like moving from dance kindergarten to the first grade. I was graduating from *Pre Bronze* (what I have been calling Klutz 1), *to Bronze 1*.Graduation requirements were simple, although I didn't think so at the time. I had to show the head instructor the basic steps of my three dances, and then on graduation day dance all three dances along with other couples. At the time I thought I was pretty good because I had gone from zilch to doing real steps and a few moves. When I look back they were all pretty basic, and I looked rather stiff in the video I viewed afterward.

Now let's do a fast forward to one year later and my ongoing mission to reconfigure myself to keep from looking like a dry, wilted beanstalk while dancing. I tried to "stand tall and erect," as my teachers directed, keeping "my head over my heart." That works when I concentrate on just that, but then when I think about the steps I wilt a little.

Nonetheless I had learned a lot in the past year, and although I didn't qualify for another graduation, my teachers set me up for a solo routine. We wanted it to be special, a little different, so my teaches chose a jazzy song called *Do You Love Me?* by The Contours. It allowed for a little play acting and drama before we went into a fast paced single time swing.

Nervous as a cat, I stepped out and pantomimed the first lyrics of the song which were spoken: *"You broke my heart"*—[my hand over my heart, as I looked down in despair]—*"cause I couldn't dance; but now . . . I'm back!"*—[I whipped around, head up, standing tall and faced my partner a several feet in front of me]— *"and I can really shake 'em down!"* [I did a quick imitation of the *Twist*.]

At that point my partner, Ali, ran out to me and we started swingin'. She was a pretty, petite young teacher who danced with effortless grace.

When we heard the lyrics go to *Do the twist, mashed potatoes,* we broke apart and started gyrating in a lively twist motion, which was a nice surprise for the audience. We then went back to some conventional moves and finally, stopped, faced the crowd as though we were about to take our bows. But instead we dropped down into a wild Twist to the music again, which the spectators weren't expecting, but they quickly recovered and gave us another big burst of applause.

I still smile when I remember my graceful partner, my raw nerves before and my elation afterwards. Now fast forward another year and I did finally graduate from Bronze 1 to Bronze 2. I'm likely to stay in the *Bronze Age* for a long time, maybe the rest of my life. But that's not a bad thing if I am still dancing until the very end. In fact, it would be a good way to go! Maybe doing the Lindy hop or the polka? Yeah!

One day at a practice party long after the above routine, I was dancing the hustle to this same song with one of my favorite teachers. We like to joke around with each other. As we hustled, the refrain *"Do You Love Me?"* was vibrant in my ears, and then I heard my partner's lusty wisecracking, "Do you love me, Harvey?

"YES, I LOVE YOU, Zoila! I yelled, then we both busted up with hilarity as we attempted to finish our dance.

This is an example of the special qualities our teachers have, and this is typical of the positive undercurrent that flows in a gathering of happy dancers.

Now settle down and see what Jeremy has to say. This is a great narrative..

Jeremy's Story

While in a conversation over the phone with my then girlfriend, we started talking about our ideal dream dates. We bounced a few off of one another and then I spoke about one that I had envisioned in my twenties: I pictured a masquerade ball, the grand ballroom, and the costumes, with everyone dancing some classical smooth dance. *How cool would it be to take to that the person you were head over heels for?!* I had never done this in my twenties because of a multitude of excuses, and I am good about rationalizing away anything. As I was then in my late thirties I was keenly aware of my tendency to talk myself out of things. I would say, "I need to have a dance partner to go." Or "I;m young. I got time to try this later." These were among a list of numerous excuses. The realization hit me that I should be dancing instead of talking about it.

I expected that I would not be very good at dancing with no prior background in it, nor did I care to watch others dance. Aside from that, I did not know what to expect and I had no assumptions going in. Turns out I was correct on my first point in that I was slow to get a grasp on many concepts, but that did not deter me.

The first place I went to learn to dance was a very new experience to me. It was difficult and I was not having too much fun, but I had no benchmark on what the experience should be. I never took any of the group lessons, as I felt I was not ready for them. But I was continuing on my progress thinking that this will get better and more fun as I learn more.

As time went on I tried a different studio that was closer to where I lived. The energy was completely different and the instructor was completely engaged in the lesson with my partner and me. I found myself laughing and learning, and in the span of a few minutes the instructor got me past things that I had been struggling with for months. My eyes were opened to a totally different atmosphere and learning experience. I was completely hooked. Even when I saw that the expense of this studio was going to be a challenge for me to afford, I still signed up and found ways to make it work.

My original goal to learn to dance is no longer the main reason I go to the studio. Yes, I do want to improve and be able to use what I have learned elsewhere, but more importantly I found the studio to be a huge positive in my life, a place that is often a de-stressor and sometimes therapeutic.

Years later this is still a positive place for me and a large reason why I continue on my lessons. Over time I have met new people and shared in many new experiences. As the years pass by many of these people have become friends and some even close friends with whom even to this day we all share in adventures, both in and outside the studio. It is the experiences and the memories that are the indelible markers of life. These are timeless happenings and things you get to keep forever, long after money and materials fade.

Chapter Fifteen
The Polka

When I started at Arthur Murray, the polka appeared to be an alien concept to my fellow students. As far as I knew, I was the only polka enthusiast, since hardly any student here had danced it. Eventually I did find a couple of polka lovers, but at first my impression was that the general crowd considered the polka a hidden bastard of the dance family.

Observing this reaction, I concluded that there were at least two things about the polka that these folks didn't seem to be aware of. One, that the basic step is easier than most of the dances they are learning, and two, that the polka beat, or rhythm, is in many songs that are not immediately recognizable as polkas. Examples are some traditional Irish tunes, Scottish bagpipe selections, country songs like Willy Nelson's *Yellow Rose of Texas, Just Because You Think You're so Pretty* by Bobby Vinton, and even commonly heard songs like *Sugar in the Morning*.

So if you hear some music that is even too fast for a Single Time Swing, chances are the polka would work, and be less tiring.

My instructors were aware that the polka was the only dance I knew before I came to Arthur Murray. That's why one of the instructors one day suggested that a polka *Demo* would be appropriate for me. A *Demo* is one way to motivate students to improve our skills and build confidence. For a demo we work with our teacher on a routine which we'll do as a solo performance before our peers.

Therefore, one day in November when I came to the dance center for a lesson, innocent and unsuspecting, the head instructor, Kate, caught me off guard when she said: "How about doing a polka demo at the Christmas dance?"

"A polka at Christmas?" I said. "I doubt it. Who ever heard of a Christmas polka?" I figured I was safe.

"Here's one," Kate said a moment later as she did a search ion her phone. "It's even called *The Christmas Polka*."

She got me.

So Kate and I worked up a routine and performed it before half my family and everybody else at the Christmas dance. This then, served as an introduction of the polka to the students at this dance center. Kudos to Kate, my dedicated teacher.

After that, Arthur Murray Folsom was no longer a polka virgin. The instructors selecting the songs started playing polkas occasionally at some of the practice parties. On one of these occasions, teacher Ronit came to me, eager to dance the polka. It was news to me that she had a background in Folk Dance, including the polka. Her polka dancing was superb, and I could see then that she had more polka knowledge than I would ever have. Eventually she worked up a polka routine with me for a demo which we performed at our Folsom center.

But the most memorable performance of this routine was at a *Spotlight* event in the ballroom of a Marriott's Hotel. Besides our large contingent of dancers from Arthur Murray Folsom, the

Carmichael center was also there in full force, as well as a few guests, including a table full of my kids, grandkid and great grandkids who had come to see me demonstrate my glorious skill, dancing my solo polka with teacher Ronit.

It was a fairly complicated routine with a lot of hand styling in coordination with the polka steps. At one point, I took off in the wrong direction doing a traveling step. "Oh, we're facing the wrong way!" I heard Ronit whisper. That threw the whole routine off.

And here is where I want to pause to share a tip with all beginning dance students: If you screw up a routine, even if it's a big mistake, *keep going* as best you can, as if nothing happened. The slogan is, *fake it until you make it!*

And that is just what we did. With Ronit's guidance we kept polkaing like we knew what we were doing. But I knew I had messed up, and was devastated. However, afterwards, as I cautiously queried for reactions, it was obvious that no one knew there had been a foul up. When I watched the video later, even though I knew better, I could detect no obvious mistakes.

At our dance center now the polka is not considered as much of a bastard step child as before. Not often, but sometimes ladies even ask, "Will you dance the polka with me? It looks fun!"

And just in case you were thinking the polka is illegal, it actually is in the Arthur Murray syllabus. Sure would be nice to have more company on the dance floor, hopping, whooping, and laughing, for the polka is a happy dance.

But the ground of ballroom dancing is not the most fertile soil for cultivating a large crop of polka dancers, so I'm trying to fertilize it. I won't tell you what I'm using. So now and then we have our moments. One day at a Saturday dance an instructor announced a polka, "For Harvey!" I'd rather it be for everybody, but some are leery of it because they perceive it as being extremely vigorous and exhausting. This is most likely my fault. There is something in my DNA that makes me want to go the limit, spin, yell, and get a little crazy. The music makes me do it; I'm not to blame. I just hope I don't look like a fired-up up soccer player dancing around, desperate to score a goal—or worse, an over zealous fan looking to kill the opponent.

So it's no wonder that people don't know that this dance can be done as sedately and calm as a waltz, albeit not as elegantly. Just watch some of those eighty and ninety-year-old folks of the polka club. They keep a smooth rhythm and don't expend surplus energy.

I wanted my dance friends to experience the ambience of an authentic polka event, so I persuaded a few of them to come with me to the *Polka Booster Club,* of which I had formerly been a member many years prior. Incredibly the same band, called *Polka Power* was playing.

This day we were treated to a typical polka party. When the first vibrant notes were sounded, the place came to life. There were divergent polka techniques, with some couples hopping happily and emitting lusty yells, while some of the others were moving with measured, not athletic, control, but were having as much fun as the more boisterous types. I couldn't refrain from pointing out to my comrades that when I yell while doing the polka at Arthur Murray, that's not me going crazy; it's a normal part of the action.

My friends seemed receptive to this new escapade, not only observing but trying out their polka dexterity. Then after a couple of polkas, the band played some waltzes, a rhumba and a tango, and my ballroom-dancing friends excelled in those before their next polka challenge.

For strangers who showed up suddenly into their circle, we were very well received and urged, "Come back again and bring more of you!"

This club comprised generally older folks than we're used to at Arthur Murray. I mentioned to a club lady that I thought it was ironic that my younger circle shied away because they considered the polka too strenuous.

"Baloney," she said. "The polka can be danced as slow and easy as any other dance!" Maybe I should take a cue from that observation.

But did I? Two months later we went back to the polka Boosters. I wasn't quite as wild and did try to include some other moves which were tamed down a bit. This time there were more of us, and the club welcomed us warmly, again urging that we return. At 6:00 p.m., as they played their last polka, it seemed to be a tradition for all to gather in front of the band to sway and clap in cadence to show *Polka Power* our appreciation for their music making.

This was the first time in many years that I had spent four hours dancing like I used to when I was younger. I'm still recovering. But it was worth it, and I'll do it again if I get a chance.

If you prefer the smooth dances, it's understandable why the polka doesn't float your boat.. But you should at least give it a shot sometime. You may even like it a little. And it's been around longer than you may think.

Today, polka is one of the few dances that originated during the nineteenth century that is still popular worldwide. Historic folklore has it that a peasant girl named Anna Slezak invented the steps. The word "pulka" is derived from the Czech phrase for "half-step," which refers to the dance pattern of lightly stepping from one foot to the other.

The polka dance was first introduced to Prague ballrooms in 1835, and it soon grew wildly popular. Polka eventually reached England and the United States by the late 1840s.

[Latest bulletin: There is a rumor that there will soon be a group class in the polka at our studio. If this happens, it will be the first time since I've been coming here.

Also, teacher Renata has been showing me some new moves to use in the polka. So . . . *the polka lives on!*]

Next, Gil's contribution shows us that even when life takes some bad turns, we can still get back on the road and keep on truckin'; or in this case, dancing.

Gil's Story

My wife of thirty-seven years passed away four years ago from lung cancer. We loved to dance, although she was not into ballroom dancing. After a period of grieving, my parents, who were avid ballroom dancers, encouraged me to get out and dance. They knew that I had enjoyed ballroom dancing when I tried it once with my wife.

So I mustered up the courage to go out and give it a try. The instructors at the dance studio were so inviting and encouraging, I decided to sign up.

However, it was not as easy as I thought it might be. There was a learning curve. As the moves got more involved, I became discouraged at times. My muscle memory was failing me. Was I getting too old for dancing? But being a lifelong learner and teacher of students, I knew that it was a process of confusion and enlightenment. I hung in there and now feel a lot more confident, although I still get confused and unsure of myself.

Besides the mechanics of dancing, I enjoy the company of wonderful people: the instructors, my dance partners, and the other men who willingly share their expertise with me.

None of the women, young or old, tall or short, say no, when I ask them to dance. One has a sense of acceptance. If I make a mistake in the dance routine, we laugh and try it again. It is a safe place to make mistakes. Shouldn't life be like that? The world would be a better place.

There are so many other benefits to dancing that I enjoy. Although I might feel tired at the end of the day, when I get to the dance studio in the evening, I feel energized and alive. I figure it must be great for my health. Also, memorizing all those dance patterns, which is the role of the leader, challenges and stimulates my mind as I process the new information.

Lastly, I have created some wonderful friendships with fellow dancers, some of whom have shared their life stories with me. Dancing is such a bonding experience.

Sometimes I encounter unexpected surprises. I was a teacher for thirty-one years, and very often run into former students. So who do I get to dance with one evening? Yes, a student I had taught when she was thirteen years old, but she is now a mom and a lot taller than she was so many years ago. I hope I gave her a passing grade!

I feel blessed and grateful for the many surprises life has given me, especially after the death of my dear wife. I miss her every day, but I am sure she is smiling and encouraging me to keep dancing, until the day we meet again and dance in the heavens.

Chapter Sixteen
Cha Cha

"Oh my God, this is impossible; I'll never learn it!"

And I was still just working on the basic step. So my steadfast instructor, Yajenny, made a diagram of the foot placements. "You can take this home and practice."

When I looked at it at home, at first it merely resembled examples of the Arabic alphabet that I had seen. But after a second study it started making sense— so I practiced—and practiced— until I got it.

But you can't just repeat the basic step over and over for the whole dance as you thumb your nose at the spectators and say, "See what I can do?" No, you have to learn some *moves,* like *her turn, crossover break, alternate turn, open break* . . . and more. This would take years!

It was months rather than years, and I was only able to pull it off because Yajenny was so dedicated and encouraging, and never gave up on me. As we practiced, her reassuring smile was always there to bolster me. Then one day she said, "You're ready."

"Ready for what?" I asked suspiciously.

"Your first cha cha demo!"

A fleeting sensation of terror struck at my heart . . . then faded. I knew it was time to run the gauntlet in front of my contemporaries.

As always, Yajenny had more confidence in me than I had in myself. But our first demo was passable, and we did two more solos after that at special dance venues.

But just because I could cha cha with my teacher, I didn't metamorphose into an Afro-Cuban dance celebrity. In fact when I danced with fellow students, I realized that leading the cha cha properly was going to be a whole new learning curve.

"Turn when I turn," I told my partner, as Yajenny looked on.

"No Harvey," she said, patiently. "You don't tell them; you lead with your body and hands. Swing their hand and start your turn and they'll know they are supposed to turn as you turn."

Unless you simply repeat endlessly what you know and nothing else, you never stop learning in the art of dance. So for us guys, learning to lead is usually phase two of any dance. As leaders, it is our responsibility to work on these skills constantly. It seems harder than what the gals have to do, huh? But be reminded that our teachers have to learn both leading and following to qualify for certification. And I've heard that there are ladies who would rather lead, and have to resign themselves to always be the followers.

The cha cha is a true Latin dance, which originated in Cuba where it evolved from the Danzon, an older form of Cuban dance. The primary difference in cha cha is the addition of a triple step that replaces the slow step in mambo/rumba. I'm much more comfortable with the cha cha now, and can even get some Cuban Motion into it, (hey hey!) but there's still plenty of room for improvement. Will I live long enough?

And my wonderful cha cha teacher, Yajenny, won't be here to see it, because, to our sorrow, but with our blessings, she left to complete her graduate work at the university. I hope she can come back and visit some day and cha cha with me.

Meanwhile, thank goodness, there are other excellent teachers here. But are they ready for old man Klutz?

Dance Move Definitions

By now you have seen the names of several dance moves, so I thought it would be helpful to describe these moves. But then it occurred to me that if you dance, you know what they are, and if you don't dance these definitions wouldn't mean squat to you. So I just decided to have a little fun with them, tongue planted firmly in cheek.

These are all bona-fide names of Arthur Murray dance moves.

CHA CHA CHASE: When she doesn't want to cha cha with you, so you have to run her down.

ALTERNATE TURN: The turn you end up doing after messing up the one you started.

ARM CHECK: An inspection to make sure you're not packing heat.

BACKHAND CHANGE: When the slight-of-hand cashier gives you back a ten instead of the twenty he owes you.

BACK ROCK: a precipitous step in reverse by an American in England as he starts to cross the street looking to the left instead of the right.

CROSSOVER BREAK: A dash across a busy intersection when the light is yellow.

PEEKABOO: Don Juan casts a devious smile at that sexy babe every time she looks at him over her dance partner's shoulder.

CROSS BODY LEAD: You step in front of that jerk who is eyeing your partner and then with a sudden action lead her clear away from him.

THE CONTINUOUS THROWOUT: When your tenants repeatedly fail to pay their rent.

CONTINUOUS THROWOUT AND LINK: She keeps kicking him out, then making up.

"So," my new teacher says, "you've learned the cha cha. What's next, the salsa?" *Salsa! Oh, my God, that is impossible; I could never learn it!* Yeah, I know, I said the same thing about the ca cha, but...

Lindy Hop

So I found an excuse to procrastinate; I'm putting the salsa in the back of the line for a while because of a scene that captivated me at a practice party: Single time swing music came blasting on with a killer rhythm and such an animated melody that it struck me just like the first time I heard a polka. I wanted to jump around with that irresistible beat but didn't know how. Then I saw a young couple that obviously did. I mean they were really hoofing it, hot and happy! It looked like they were doing a little hop, alternating with a kick— yes, they were kicking! The couple was well synchronized to the music and each other. It was very energetic and surely satisfied that urge that comes with such a hot piece of music. I had heard of the Lindy hop, but this is the first time I had ever seen it.

[The Lindy hop, named after Lindbergh, is a partner dance that originated in the 1920's and 30's in Harlem, New York. The Dance includes footwork borrowed from the Charleston and Tap.

"Shorty" George Snowden, an African American and his partner Mattie Purnell invented the Lindy Hop, and claim that they called it *The hop* before Lindbergh did his hop across the Atlantic.]

Watching the Lindy hop for the first time was a thrilling experience for me. I loved it and all I could think of was—I want to do it! So my next lessons were the *Lindy hop*.

To do this dance you alternate a *back rock,* then two forward, low kicks, knees slightly bent. After you get the basic down you go into a variety of swing patterns. A couple of advanced moves adapted for the Lindy, are the *Charleston,* a backward kick, and the *Jig,* a series of kicks without the back rock, the balboa and others that I have not learned.

So I started to learn the Lindy hop, but was disappointed that it was a polka *deja vu*—meaning that hardly any of my dancing contemporaries were interested in it! Yes, it is also strenuous like the polka, so is that the hangup? Or because it's not smooth or elegant? But how about a little variety in your dancing card? You say you want exercise? Hey, this is your chance!

Most of my colleagues here seem to consider the Lindy Hop as more fitting for the "younger set." Don't they know this is a way to stay young themselves? So now I'm constantly on the lookout for more Lindy kickers as well as polka hoppers. Looks like I'll have to create them myself.

My devious tactic for achieving this is to request a single time swing which lends itself to the Lindy as well as the swing. The unsuspecting, good natured lady I invite to dance assumes we'll dance the single time, so I have to be creative. We start out with a minute of swing steps, then I suggest, as though the idea just occurred to me, "Do you want to try a little Lindy hop?" Then we shift into the kicking, as I reward her with my biggest and most impish smile.

The last time I employed this tactic, the lady started protesting, "Oh, I don't know how."

"Don't worry," I assured her, "I'll teach you. Back rock as usual, then two little kicks, like this!"

So, chuckling, she tried to get in the game, and did pretty well for her first time. I have hopes that she will fall in love. No, not with me, but with the Lindy hop. That didn't happen, but since she chuckled I thought at least she had gotten a kick out of it.

Since there are relatively few who want to submit themselves to the infelicitous Lindy hop, and I can't force the issue, I guess I'll have to resign myself to a shortage of this particular discipline. But I'm still on the hunt for livewire lady Lindy hoppers.

Do you wonder why an old *over-the-hill reprobate* like me wants to do these high energy dances? The answer is because when I'm doing them I feel so happy. And because I can . . . still . . . for now.

More Ways to Look at Dance Moves

FIFTH POSITION: Yeah, and you're lucky to have that after flirting with your boss's wife.

GRAPEVINE: When you get so confused you can't make up your mind which way to turn.

HANDSHAKE TURN: You shake hands with your opponent to get him off guard, then use a quick Jiu jitsu move to turn him on his ass.

HEAD LOOP: The result of three or more Margaritas.

HESITATION: You really want to ask that sexy chick to dance, but you're so chicken you freeze.

INSIDE TURN: Okay, this is just between you and me.

RIGHT SIDE SWEETHEART: My boyfriend is so totally right side dominated that I know he won't stray.

THE LEFT SIDE SWEETHEART: The one you're trying to keep secret from the right side sweetheart.

LINK: You've decided to go steady.

You're never too old or too young to start dancing. But I wish I had started as early as Christopher did; even if I didn't have his natural talent.

Kristopher's Story

My dance story begins when I was fifteen, and my grandparents bought me ten lessons at the local Arthur Murray studio for Christmas. Now I had always been interested in ballroom dancing after hearing all of my parents' stories of their social dancing, but when I held the gift card in my hand I could feel my little dreams gradually come to life.

When that first blast of cold air hit me as I opened the studio door for the first of thousands of times, I wasn't sure if I would like dancing. What if my grandparents wasted their money on something that I would hate? What if I just wasn't good at it? What if people laughed at me for dancing? My fears ran rampant through my mind until I finally got to dancing. Almost immediately I fell entirely in love. Every step I took and every step I continue to take brings me more enjoyment than anything else I could do.

Over a year later I'm still dancing. In September of 2018 I participated in my first competition as a beginner and won every category, and now I am hoping to go to the next level in my next competition.

Dancing has brought me so much joy over time that it's hard to believe that I ever considered not going. It has taught me to have courage, to never give up no matter how hard the situation, (or steps for that matter), might be. But most of all it has taught me to not doubt my abilities. Overall dancing has shown me a new perspective to life. One that is full of light and music to the point where there just isn't time to be sad. I look forward to dancing in my future and maybe turning it into a career.

Chapter Seventeen
Saint Patrick's Day

What I did that day was totally unplanned and afterward I kind of wish I hadn't done it, as I had gotten myself into a box.

It was 2018, St. Paddy's Day, and we had a violinist here at the old folk's home. He was good, and the Irish tunes he was playing were so peppy and buoyant that I felt compelled to rise up out of my seat and move to the beat. It seemed about right for the Lindy hop so I started rocking while we were eating lunch right there in the dining room with everyone gawking, and probably thinking, "What the hell is that idiot doing?"

Surprisingly, they loved it and were sure it was an Irish Jig. I had copious compliments for days afterwards. Actually they liked it *too much*, and the following year, February, 2019, it occurred to me: *they will be expecting me to do it again.*

So be it, I said, but this time I want to dance it with a partner. But who at my Arthur Murray center would be willing to do the Lindy hop with me? There must be at least one risk taker who's willing to give it a go.

First, I prevailed on my Arthur Murray instructors to help with my search. So one day an instructor hailed me. "Hey, there's this nice girl, she's fifteen, who loves to dance the Lindy. Her parents can drop her off and you can do the routine with her."

So back to the *more-suitable*-younger-crowd syndrome, huh? What is this a self fulfilling prophecy? As much as I appreciated the willingness of that sweet little girl, I really wanted a grown up lady dancing with me.

Then I thought of fellow-student, Kris, who is one of a very few who likes to polka with me. Maybe she'd be up for this Lindy gig.

"Sure, sounds fun," she said, "but I don't know the Lindy."

"Well, we have over a month to get ready."

"Okay," she said, and signed up for a Lindy lesson.

All right, I thought, *we're on the way!*

Then I was told about another student, Carolyn, a gold rated dancer, who excelled in the Lindy, and had indicated an interest in performing it with me. That's wonderful! But what about Kris? I appreciated her willing spirit and was not going to dis-invite her.

I talked to the ladies and they were fine with both of them participating. The routine would be repeated in different sections of the dining room, and they could just take turns dancing with me. What's not to like about that? Later, my friend Yuriko offered to come and support us any way she could. Things are looking good!

Then Murphy's Law imposed its first strike: *The violinist is not going to be here this St. Patrick's Day.* Our Irish music, the original motivation—gone! There lie my best laid plans, shot in the ass! Even though this meant I was off the hook, no expectations now, I felt let down. I had gotten myself and the ladies all revved up and now we're hanging in limbo. So I went Irish jig searching in iTunes.

I found several nice Irish Jigs, but only one had a tempo fast enough for the Lindy hop. Another was a full orchestra, classic Irish, that was so rousing, I knew I had to use it some way. It had a beat too slow for Lindy, but perfect for a polka. Just hearing it prompted spontaneous body motion or clapping to the beat. I felt a noncompliant sensation invade my psyche: This Irish celebration was about to be infiltrated by polka power. I hoped to sneak it in so they wouldn't notice this foreign element.

I had noticed that in the last few measures of this energizing piece, the orchestra sped up to a perfect Lindy tempo, so I devised a routine that would start with the polka and finish with what looked like the Irish jig, and this would be our finale.

My program would include several people. First Carolyn and I would do the Lindy steps masquerading as Irish jigs. Then, Kris and I would do the polka, then yielding to Yuriko and my friend Andre doing the single time swing, and then Carolyn and I would wow them with a very fast Lindy hop when the music sped up at the end.

Then strike two of Murphy's Law hit us: Carolyn had come down with the flu, so our star was out of the game. Then I heard through a mutual friend that Kris had some doubts about her part because she hadn't had a chance to practice with the music we picked.

Then strike three: Management here had promised to download and broadcast our music in the dining room that day, but could not download the exhilarating full orchestra piece we wanted for our Finale. But then Kris, bless her, called and said, "Send me the music and I'll see you tomorrow at the dance and we'll practice!" That night she brought ear pods and had the music on her phone. That way we could hear our music and dance our thing while the others were dancing to cha cha and everything else.

Our program was intact again, with Kris, Yuriko, Andre and me. Then strike four came down on me. Yuriko, poor lady, called to inform me that she was sick too. But we had invested too much to give up now, so the day before the event, Teresa graciously consented to take part. Also, at the last minute we were able to transmit the missing full-orchestra, dynamic tune from Kris's phone to the PA system in the dining room.

And so it happened: Kris and I did the first two Lindy hop pieces, and then we all danced to the electrifying strain of the full-orchestra. Our aged audience, usually subdued, was clapping and shouting their approval, so we were all having fun. Jeremy and Hoeun were there in support and to video us, as was my son, Will. I am very grateful to all of those involved, because without their tenacity, this memorable event would not have come to fruition.

Usually when a person is exposed to dancing, it seems to get in their blood. Let's read about Christina's journey back to her love of dance.

Christina's Story

Why I started dancing? Well, I've always danced, but somehow along the way I stopped. As time went on, life got in the way: the job, the responsibilities, trying to keep up with everything. I knew I really needed to get back to it. I was looking for an adult ballet class, but I was too tired to go after work, so I never quite made it.

Then on a sunny weekend afternoon, walking through a wine and art festival, there was a booth that had a banner: *Arthur Murray Dance Studio*. Anything with the word *dance* in it will have me walking up to it! No one was at the table, and it was actually quite barren with a simple sign-up sheet for a free private lesson, and I thought, "why not"! I had no idea what to expect. I received a call the next day, and I booked a private lesson, specifically requesting an expert in Latin dancing.

My first lesson: I sat in the lobby of the studio feeling completely out of my element, a stranger, whilst there was a hustle and bustle of people going in and out, chatting, scheduling, and dancing. I was introduced to a very nice dancing instructor, and I had a very nervous, but great first lesson. I signed up for a month of dancing to start, and I went back the same week for another lesson. Driving home from my second session, I felt a surge of happiness! I could breathe again! I had no idea how my life had shifted and how badly my soul needed to *dance*.

I haven't stopped since. And now I know that when I need a break from life, when life gets tough and shadow peaks over me, I just need to dance!

Chapter Eighteen
The Salsa

Here's a move I mastered early on:
CHICKEN SCRATCH: What I looked like I was doing when I was trying to learn the basic salsa step.

I still viewed the salsa as a difficult dance and didn't see how I could ever learn it because the moves seemed counterintuitive to my style of dancing. Some love the salsa, and others shy away from it. But the overriding factor is that the salsa is the *most popular Latin dance in the world, so* I can no longer dis it, dang it!

To begin with, the footwork is tricky. The foot that's not stepping is supposed to be "on base", momentarily stationary. For several months I was doing a dance that I called the salsa, but undoubtedly it was an adulteration of this proud Latin tradition.

Here's what happened at a practice party:

"You're supposed to be moving forward and backward," she said. *Oh, damn, I thought I was supposed to stay on base.*

At my next lesson I demonstrated my salsa footwork. "Oh . . . yeah," my teacher Ronit said, hesitating. I think she was trying to hide her dismay.

"I see a couple of things we can work on."

She stuck a couple of short duct tape strips on the floor, and had me stand on them. "This is where you start." She explained that when each foot steps on those spots they should remain stationary while the other foot is making its move. So I did my usual step sequence and those insubordinate dogs of mine that were supposed to stay still were shuffling like a lost chicken. Man, what a hard habit to break!

After some practice to get the feel of it, she advised me to practice like that at home. So I stuck some bright yellow duct tape strips on the carpet in my little studio apartment. This caused some consternation to my poor little housekeeping girl the next time she vacuumed. She's a nice little lady and also thought my trike battery looked like a bomb, but did not report that or the yellow duct tape to my landlords, so she was cool.

The duct tape technique helped my salsa. When I went back to my lesson, Ronit was pleased with my improvement. The only way I could keep the jumpy feet stationary was with knee action in the moving steps. That turned out to be a bonus because it effected the desired Cuban motion. (hip action).

But the salsa timing is the toughest bugaboo to master. With most dances I'm usually right with the rhythm, but in the salsa I get off at times because I can't hear the beat distinctly. It's an eight count beat but the numbers four and eight are pauses. So the count is one-two-three—five-six-seven—. When I get off and try to catch up I must look like I'm playing hopscotch instead of dancing the salsa.

At another dance party I got into trouble again. I was trying to perform a *crossover break*. "Oh, no," my dance partner said, "Not so fast, you're rushing it!" That is one of my usual sins. My teacher,

Brandi, told me that she was tempted to get a T-shirt made that says, *Slow Down, Jones!*

Being corrected by your partner is a confidence crusher. But I guess a bruised ego is better than committing the same crime repeatedly without knowing what your were doing wrong. Besides, my parters are just trying to help me, and I respect them for that.

I took my sad-salsa sob story to my teacher, Brandi "I don't get salsa," I lamented, "My salsa sucks!"

"What you want to listen for are the *pulses,* Brandi explained." Then she played some salsa and I heard it: four pulses, or measures of music. I was starting to catch it.

I realized then that I'm not the only one who has trouble with salsa timing, because someone has actually invented a machine to help with this very thing. It's called the *Salsa Beat Machine.* "Listen to this." Brandi went to the console and a square diagram came up showing all the instruments of salsa music. Then she clicked something and the music started. A voice was repeating in cadence with each pulse:"One-three-five-seven . . ."

Wow, a machine to keep us from hop scotching the salsa beat. Brandi sent me that link so I could practice with it at home.

A week later during my next lesson I was practicing my salsa step, keeping one foot in place and knee action in the other leg which brought about that *Cuban motion.* "Look at Harvey moving those hips!" Brandi yelled to Wesley, who was there with his student. Wesley then came up to me. "I was just telling my student how great you are doing," he said.

Then they decided I should dance with Wesley's female student. All I did was initiate the simple lady's turn which I had done successfully many times, as it is the most basic move. But this time my brain suffered some sort of short circuit, commonly called a brain fart, and I did it wrong.

"Oh, let's try that again," Brandi said, with a slight frown. So I repeated the mistake and we got off the count. Then as Brandi was consoling the lady whom I had wronged, Wesley approached me and said calmly, "She's supposed to turn on the five . . . you had her turn on the three." I knew that. I had always started the turn on the five—except today. Am I still jinxed with the salsa? I hope not.

Earlier in this book I suggested that we should laugh at our mistakes. I did not feel like laughing that day—but I'm laughing now. And my fervent hope is that this gaffe will be my last laugh of this type.

SALSA COIN DROP: You're a Cuban Motion machine doing a hot Salsa when your change starts falling out of the hole in your pocket.

[Salsa represents a mix of Latin musical genres, but its primary component is Cuban dance music. The roots of salsa originated in Eastern Cuba (Santiago de Cuba, Guantanamo) from the Cuban *Son* (about 1920) and Afro-Cuban dance (like Afro-Cuban rumba].

So,—can you do these moves properly?

MAGIC LEFT TURN: When a guy impulsively hangs a hard left and ends up by a sparkling pool with a host of scantily clad young maidens.

OUTSIDE TURN: Happy Harry gets excited and turns her so far away that she ends up outside in the cold.

OPEN BREAK: when a couple has a noisy argument in front of all their friends and both walk away in different directions muttering obscenities.

PATTY CAKE: An elegant Waltz pattern until some good ol' boys stole it and turned it into a boisterous *HIGH FIVE!*

PROMENADE: Manly Stud resists *Cuban Motion* because he's afraid hip movements make him look effeminate so he quits his dance lesson and takes a walk to the nearest bar.

ELVIS SWIVELS: Manly Stud's teacher gives him this assignment as punishment for walking out of his lesson.

THROWOUT AND RIGHT HAND RELEASE: In retribution, Manly Stud effects an aggressive throwout, lets go and his teacher ends up in the next neighborhood. (Manly Stud is not a very nice person.)

PROMENADE CHECK: That's when you spy on your foxy girl friend who says she's just "going for a walk."

PROGRESSIVE STEP: If you're a Republican you'll have fits trying to get this one right.

RIGHT HANDED THROWOUT: You shake hands with your tenant as you say how sorry you are to evict him.

Chapter Nineteen
The Four Stages of Learning

Posted by Juan de Dios Garcia on his blog of November 11th of 2016. Juan de Dios is the owner of two Arthur Murray Dance Centers in Northern California.

THE STAGES OF LEARNING

1. INITIAL STAGE

This is the beginning stage where you first learn the dance or step. In the beginning, everything is new and exciting. Kind of like learning to drive a car. You don't know what to do, but you know you want to get out on the road and give it a shot. The great thing here is, the excitement, newness of learning different patterns, how to move your body and learning about the whole world of dance, keeps your mind off of anything in your way.

2. AWKWARD STAGE

Eventually you learn more and pass stage one and go to stage two. Here, you quickly realize that you maybe need more time to get this stuff down. That's when your body is taking time to learn and things start to feel awkward. You know this stage well. This is when you feel like your learning isn't so much learning and you start to question if you really are learning to dance or not. Trust me! You are learning to dance, your body just takes longer to learn than your head. Stick with it and trust that there is another stage to get to.

3. CONSCIOUS STAGE

If you stick with it long enough, you reach the conscious stage. This is where you feel like you have it, but you still have to think about it. Kind of like driving. At this stage, it would be easy to drive, but you still have to remember to signal and stop completely at a red light (not the California roll). Dancing can be fun, but you still have to think about what move you have to do next, or worry about other people on the floor. This is where muscle memory is being built, so it may take time before getting out of this stage.

4. NATURAL STAGE

Finally, you made it to the last stage. The Natural Stage! This is where dancing becomes easy and flows from one move to the next. It feels . . . Natural. Like you don't necessarily need dance lessons anymore, but do it because you love it. Now when people say the words "They're just a natural born dancer." You can say, "It's learned."

ONE LAST THING

The Stages of Learning are a constant and never ending process. As long as you keep learning, you will always have a learning process and another stage to go through. Most importantly, don't get discouraged. Know that every dancer (including your instructors), however good they are, were once in your very uncomfortable, self-conscious type shoes. Just remember, that when you're feeling down, it's probably your body taking time to learn and/or you are about to breakthrough to the next level. Just keep moving. Just keep Dancing!

Chapter Twenty
Blind Invitations

With my poor vision, I sometimes have a problem zeroing in on an appropriate dance partner. It doesn't help that at the practice parties the lights are dimmed. That's supposed to make it more exotic, romantic, and mysterious, you know. (And make it harder to see each others' mistakes?)

It is indeed often mysterious to me. I see a form standing on the side, watching. The form is wearing a pretty dress so I figure she must be female, unless one of our instructors is in drag, so I make my way over to her. "Would you like to dance?"

"Oh . . . okay," she giggles. I can tell she's uncomfortable. Now I see why. She looks to be about fourteen, here with her family, not expecting to be dancing with a great grandfather. Yeah, I know, I said I'm only as old as the girl I'm dancing with; but I don't enjoy embarrassing poor little girls. And I'm not trying to be as young as fourteen.

Or I may go to the other extreme and invite a lady who is here to watch her granddaughter, and hobbles around with a cane—which I don't notice. I can tell by the glare she gives me that she desires to dance with this character that's in her face as much as she wants to be plastered across the grill of a speeding Mercedes.

An instructor observes me in my dance-partner-searching mode. "Why don't you ask those ladies sitting across on the other side?

"There are spare women across the hall?" I exclaim in surprise. If they are clear across this dimly lit dance floor, they might as well be in North Platte, Nebraska, as far as my weak peepers are concerned. My only recourse is to walk around, like Mr. Magoo, staring into faces, hoping I don't look like a livestock inspector.

But these gaffes don't happen to me all the time. What I really like is when a lady invites me to dance. So I slip a cue to my dance teachers and others to encourage the ladies to invite me because they can locate me easier than I can locate them.

And I'm sure as hell not so blind that I go around touching and feeling to make sure they're female.

My best recourse for finding a dance partner is to stay out in the middle of the floor after a dance has just finished until some nice lady comes along and picks me off for the next dance. Doesn't always work, but it's better than blind lurching in the realm of shadowy forms.

Okay, I laid that last part on a bit thick. But seriously, ladies, here's something for you.

ODE TO MY DANCE PARTNERS
(Adapted from the song *Diana)*

You're so young and I'm so old
But all my partners you are gold

I don't care that we're years apart
Your allure is high, it's off the chart
You and I will waltz, then fly
Then you'll move on to the next lucky guy

Oh, please come again, my partners

The pleasure I get from just your smile
That, to me, makes the wait worthwhile
Oh, my partners, can you not see?
I'll hold my frame if you come to me

What enjoyment I get when you move to my cue
That's why it's so nice, dancing with you

Oh, please, my partners, come dance with me

Sometimes I'm off, I make a mistake
Will you please forgive me, for goodness sake?
I admire you, I respect you, you are the best
And when dancing with you, I feel like I'm blessed

Please, my partners, come dance with me

The Stages of Learning Oddball Dance Moves

SHE/HE TURN: Finally—Gender equality!

SUGAR PUSH: You're trying to lose weight so you give that double bowl of ice-cream a big shove away from you.

WAIST ROLL: A coil of fat around your middle that you can't get rid of.

SHOULDER ROLL: The same as a waist roll except you can tell people that the bulge on your shoulder is muscle, not fat.

SWEETHEART: Save this one until you're dancing with that lady you want to get close to, then use it repeatedly.

TUCK: What you have to do with all that excess skin after losing ninety pounds.

UNDERARM TURN: Followers, before you commit to this you may want to make sure he has bathed and applied his deodorant.

WALKS AND POINTS: What a guide does when he takes people to see historic sites.

Chapter Twenty-One
Fickle Eyeballs

This happened just once since I started taking lessons, and that was enough, because it was perplexing. That one evening my visual acuity was not only abnormally clear, it was selective.

I had asked a young lady in her twenties to dance the rhumba. She was all smiley, sweet, and bright faced. I couldn't help but notice her very tight T-shirt. Oh my . . . and she had a . . . very . . . let's say . . . a prominent chest. Okay, so what?! Why should I even be aware of that? I'm a great grandfather, for crud's sake! She's a healthy, innocent child. Well . . . in her twenties. Of course I don't know for a fact how innocent she is. But as far as I'm concerned, she's just a sweet, innocent young lady and deserves my respect. Why should I even notice her . . . upper body ampleness. It irritates me that I do. I have no inappropriate urges or emotions. I respect all these ladies here, younger or older, and enjoy dancing and socializing with them.

I once heard a mother of a teenage daughter say that she thought testosterone should be a *Controlled Substance* among teenaged boys. Maybe she has a point. But that has nothing to do with this situation. For me that was way back in the past. Any little bit of my juvenile testosterone that may have held on has surely ebbed away long ago.

I wish God would explain to me why She's allowing me to be aware of these feminine attributes when I'm not trying to see them and have no intention of dilly dallying around. But if She wouldn't even tell me why She started producing so many tall women, She darn sure won't elucidate this issue for my benefit. I suppose the pragmatic answer is that I am a heterosexual, human male with blood still moving in his veins.

The good thing is that this only happens with a complete stranger. So I'll get this gal's name, and then chit-chat for a moment and she will be converted in my mind from bosom to person. Then everything will be back to normal.

In my distraction, I had almost forgotten which dance we were doing. Oh, yeah, the rhumba. I'll just keep my eyes on her face or over her shoulder. We'll be fine.

More Tips on Mastering Those Zany Moves

SECOND POSITION: You're vice-president, only one more step to go, so get ready to do some serious mud-slinging and trash-talking.

SWING STEP: A sudden evasive step to the left you have to make to avoid stepping in the dog poop.

SHADOW ROCKS: What you look for on a hot, sunny day when you're hiking and want to find a place to sit and rest.

LADY'S FAN: Happy Hannah accelerated her hip swivel so much she created a breeze.

TRIPLE LADY'S FAN: Hannah's two sisters join her in the frenzied jive.

PUZZLE: Any new move my teachers are trying to teach me.

Chapter Twenty-Two
Western Swing Revisited

It's time to check out a different dance venue. I'm curious to see how I'll do after all these lessons. A good gauge would be Western Swing that my old skiing buddy, Monte, took me to.

At Arthur Murray I'd been practicing a little country two step with Gail, so I invited her to accompany me.

"Well, here you are again, what a nice surprise!" Candy exclaims, as she gives me a big hug. She made us feel welcome as soon as we showed up. "Would you like to sit at our table? I'll round up some chairs."

Candy is a big-boned, personable gal, who likes to do things in a big way. Of all the tables in the room, only her table was decorated with a nice tablecloth and a big cake, plates, spoons, and birthday cards because she's always observing someone's birthday with a celebration right here.

Candy was attired neatly in a full skirt and sporting a big, bright red cowboy hat. She is authentic, because she used to be a rodeo performer, a barrel racer, and roper, I think. But unfortunately she is now curtailed due to physical ailments, and even has to limit her dancing to the slow ones. But she is spirited and loquacious and the gentlemen still come seek her out for dances and conversation.

The other lady there, named Gail, coincidentally the same name as my companion that day, gave us another friendly greeting and some more hugs.

Also present was the New Zealander, Pat, who had once given me a dance lesson in Monte's garage. I did poorly enough that it could have brought her to tears, but fortunately she laughed instead.

The cordial reception by these ladies made me feel a little guilty that I had not come back sooner, but my dancing skills were so inferior that I was ashamed to make an appearance until I had at least learned enough so I wouldn't embarrass myself.

After meeting the rest of the folks at the table, Gail and I did our version of the country two-step, and also managed to sneak in a hustle and even a *faux* polka that had a polka rhythm even though it wasn't recognized as a polka.

Of course Monte was there, charming all the ladies as usual, with his smooth dancing and smart-assed witticisms. He has a talent for making remarks that sound insulting, but the ladies think it's cute. For example, one gal was complaining that her back hurt. Monte said, "Well if you hadn't spent so much time on your back when you were young you wouldn't have that problem!" That earned him a little slap and a giggle, because they love him and know him for the good guy that he really is.

Another time a lady joked that she knew where Viagra was available cheap, in case he was interested, and Monte said, "Viagra hell, my ankle is already so damn stiff I can hardly dance on it!"

Gail and I watched the two-stepping western swingers to check their techniques. Coming from Arthur Murray we were used to a wider variety of dance styles, but these people provided their own variety in the two-step with moves I couldn't identify. It looked fun, but would take me a while to learn them, and I had all I could handle trying to improve my ongoing ballroom skills.

The ambience at Western Swing was informal and upbeat, like most dancing venues. One old guy, a complete stranger, came up to me: "I'm older than you are!" he declared for no reason I could think of except that he thought I qualified to be a member of the over-the-hill gang.

"Well," I answered, "maybe you're older, but not much."

"I'm ninety," he boasted.

"Okay, in a few months I'll turn ninety myself."

"You will?" he said, apparently surprised. But soon recovered, and said, "My doctor couldn't believe that I'm ninety I'm in such good shape."

"That's great!"

"My other doctor is dead!" he affirmed.

[Ah, the George Burns syndrome, I thought: *When they asked George what his doctors said about all his smoking and drinking Burns said "My doctors are dead."*]

Before we left Western Swing that day a lady approached me: "Hi, Barney," she said, "I see you've improved your dancing skills." She was my first, trial dance partner from *danceparnters.com,* the one whose skills were more advanced than mine, so I had to terminate the partnership. I was pleased to see that she had continued dancing, and even had a partner there and seemed happy. I appreciated her making the effort to come over and say hello.

After some goodbye hugs and promises to come back, we left the western swingers and it was clear to me that there was still a lot more to learn about the country two step.

Chapter Twenty-Three
Our Professionals

I arrived early at the dance center for my lesson and all the teachers were involved in their usual Staff Development project. Today's activity was a rehearsal of a routine for the Nor-Cal-San Jose District Showcase.

At other times, when they are not teaching, I see them perfecting new steps and techniques, or planning a group class that they're going to teach.

They are our teachers, first and foremost, but the role that they play is wider than I realized. First, before teaching any class at the studio, they must undergo preliminary instruction to certify. Then *Real Time* Training continues daily and weekly including business, communication, and culture training.

They also attend District-Dance-Conference Training every summer, two area trainings a year, National, and World events (Dance-O-Ramas / Competition), and local events like a Sacramento Spotlight Party.

Our instructors sometimes have the opportunity to accompany students abroad to special dance events at other Arthur Murray centers.

Occasionally the studio will do an event for the instructors that will just focus more on community bonding. But what we students like the best is their professional shows done just for us at in-studio events, such as the performance that delighted us at the 2018 Christmas party. The entire teaching staff portrayed a family's humorous tribulations on Christmas Eve. It was so well done and so stirring that we rose in unison to give them a standing ovation.

Chapter Twenty-Four
To London To Dance

July, 2018: "No, I can't possibly go to London," I insisted. "I don't have that kind of money, I have to go to the bathroom too often to be with a group, and I'm too old to endure a ten hour flight."

October 9, 2018: "This Virgin Atlantic aircraft is huge," I extolled, "and I think I'm going to like this premium seating. Thanks, Kate, for helping me get through the airport." She was looking out for me like she was my daughter. I poked aimlessly at the TV screen until Kate showed me how to access a movie. I had a beer and then watched a movie while enjoying a good dinner. If you have to endure a ten our flight, this is the way to do it.

Kate is the Arthur Murray Folsom franchise owner and teacher, and her husband, Bobby, was going along as a dance judge. There were three other students besides myself, and two other teachers. One reason I came is because I liked them all, and we did mesh well together. They ranged in age from the twenties to sixty—and then me, eighty-nine, legally blind, and keeping my bad eyes on the nearest restroom. But these companions all seemed to understand and were very accommodating.

The story I had concocted to impart to anyone watching was that these youngsters had to bring the old man along as he (I) was too senile to leave at home alone. "Are we in London yet?" I would ask as they were shepherding me through security in San Francisco.

During the flight I got up and walked, went to the restroom, settled down, went to the restroom, closed my eyes, went to the restroom—sat down, and failed to get any sleep. Then before I knew it, they were serving breakfast and getting ready to land.

To get through Customs in London, Kate took advantage of traveling with a *Special-Assistance* passenger, by having Bobby, herself, and I take the *fast track*.

"He's ninety-two and needs assistance," Kate told the agent. *Ninety-two?* I thought. *Isn't eighty-nine old enough? And she didn't even mention anything about the senile part.*

The agent studied us. "What's your relationship?"

"We're . . . friends," answered Kate. The agent leveled a blank stare at us.

"Dance friends," I added, as Bobby hung in the background.

The agent returned our passports and we were free. We got through before our friends who had been ahead of us. Then we all took the shuttle to the big city to begin our London adventure.

England—A Foreign Country

The fact that I was no longer home was reinforced when I started to take my first English shower that evening. I was confronted with four gleaming, silver-like, round knobs. But there was no shower head in sight.

With some trepidation I turned the top mystery knob and was immediately jolted by a burst of cold water pouring on my head from somewhere high above. I looked up to see a ten-inch-diameter sprinkler head, flush with the ceiling, some distance above the tub. I had a choice of a cloud burst or a horizontal pipe pointed at my chest like the barrel of a rifle. They speak English here, but it's still a foreign country.

Gallivanting with The Brits

The first night in London we went to an Indian restaurant where Kate treated us all to dinner to celebrate Bobby's birthday. Afterwards, most of those young bloods wanted to go out and do some exploring. Sounded fun, but my accumulated years had given me enough common sense to realize that after that sleepless ten-hour flight, I knew I had to get my rest, so Kate and Bobby got a taxi and saw me back to the hotel. The next morning when I heard that my buddies didn't get back until 1:00 a.m. I was glad I had refrained.

Thursday, October 11, we started the day with our first English breakfast. I was apprehensive that it might consist merely of Scones and tea. No. The buffet offered three choices of eggs, besides beans, broccoli, spinach, little red baked potatoes, bacon, sausage, and the English breakfast special, little sautéed mushrooms. Also a choice of cereals, rice, fruit and juice. I loaded my plate up and went back for more. And, thank goodness, coffee was the popular drink, not tea.

After breakfast we took the underground, *The Tube,* to get started on our city tour. Gail used to live in London so she knew how to get around on the Tube, where to get off, and which train to change to. I followed my gang around like a puppy.

The Dancing Americans

To get down to the trains we had to descend via long escalators. I've gotten irritated on escalators in the U.S. because I wanted to walk up or down, but the American dolts just stood in the way so I couldn't get by. But in London the rule is to stand on the right to allow the walkers a clear path. All of my group stood obediently on the right. As I watched some of the Brits scurrying up and down the stairs I told myself that the next time I would walk instead of stand, even if my group remained standing.

But even if these nice people I was with didn't fancy running up and down escalators, that didn't mean they weren't energetic and full of fun. They horsed around and danced everywhere they went: in the hallway to the underground, or on the platform waiting for the train, or outside to the music of a street musician.

If you ever go to London, don't mis the *London Eye*. It's an unbelievably, gigantic ferris wheel. It's called *The Eye* because when you're in it, you can see *everything*.

When we got to the bridge over the Thames River close to *The Eye*, we took photos and danced. I can say that Gail and I danced the polka on the Westminster Bridge over the River Thames to a peppy bagpipe tune.

The gigantic ferris wheel they call the *London Eye* doesn't have mere seats like a carnival ferris wheels, but rather glass encased bubbles the size of small rooms. Once inside, we gazed out the windows, mesmerized by the incredible views of this big English city. And we danced the salsa in this bubble, while the other passengers regarded us quizzically.

Superheroes and An English Tea

After our dance high in The Eye, we started walking back to catch the underground again, but the fun wasn't over yet. We came upon a British cultural icon, one of those red phone *boxes,* or booths, as we would say. That gave these creative gals an idea for what Kate called a "production."

Here's the scene: Two girls (Gail and Deanna) are attacked by two villains (Brandi and Wesley). Clark Kent (Rustin) sees them and rushes into the phone booth to change. You can see him spinning, mimicking a quick clothes change. Off camera, he exits and I enter, rustle around as though changing, then I exit, flex my muscles and go beat the villains away and save the girls.

Then *after* hanging out for a bit by Buckingham Palace, we went to our scheduled *Tea*. Very English indeed. Lunch, beer, wine, champagne, but not too much as we had an important event to attend that night.

The Royal Albert Hall

The occasion was to be a formal event, suit and tie (or bolo in my case). "The Royal Albert Hall," Kate announced to our cab driver. I got the feeling that this destination must be especially distinguished. And it was. The Royal Albert Hall opened in 1871, and has served as a venue for the world's leading artists. While it looks impressively massive from the outside, the inside is even more awesome: several stories high with tier after tier of seats, one row above the other. I was thinking that this must be what it's like to be in the most famous opera house in the world, *La Scala*, in Milan, Italy. But later I learned that La Scala's seating capacity is only 2030, compared to 5,212 here in Royal Albert Hall where we were about to take our seats.

We found them up in the thin air, and I lamented that I hadn't brought my binoculars. We were here to watch the World Championships of Latin Dances, and they were spectacular. Even though I couldn't see the detail, I could tell how precise and graceful the contestants were, gliding and twirling across the dance floor with dips and other moves so smooth they looked like they were skating.

At intermission the public was invited to go down and dance on the same floor the artists had just vacated. A horde of eager dance enthusiasts flooded onto the floor until it was jammed, shoulder to shoulder. *I'm not going down there,* I thought. I saw Gail and Brandi on the way down. *Yeah, those live wires, they would get in the middle of it.* Then Kate stood up and took my hand. "Let's go down and dance!" So she and I and Bobby snaked our way down through the multitudes.

Despite the packed dance floor, it was fun and exciting. There were all kinds of people and languages, some doing the designated dance, some not. I looked around and saw the rest of my gang out there too. No shirkers in this group!

At one point Gail and I were trying to do a fox trot. It's a traveling dance, and we weren't able to travel. So Brandi stepped in and started running interference for us, with her arm out making a way for us. Even that was slow, so she cashed in on my visual impairment. "Please," she said, "He can't see, so can you let them by?" We managed to make the complete revolution of that huge arena. What fun! And now I can say that I danced at the renowned Royal Albert Hall in London!

Escalator Games and More Sight Seeing

By the time I got to bed after leaving the Royal Albert Hall it was 1:00 a.m. That's really late for this fastidious old habit-keeper who usually tucks himself in by 10 p.m. But with this evening's experience, I considered it a luxury.

Friday, October 12 was another free day, and after another big breakfast we headed for the Tube again. This time as soon as we got on that long escalator, I hustled down the steps as fast as I could. My supportive friends let loose with a chant,"Har-vey, Har-vey." Rustin and Bobby also decided to break away and we three *high fived* at the bottom. The English spectators probably thought, *Ah, these crazy Americans are actin' a bit daft, dancin' on the underground platform and rushin' down the stairway like they're runnin' away from their old lady.*

Later in the day Rustin, Bobby, and I had kind of a race coming back up the escalator.My traveling companions must have been thinking: *We were nice enough to bring this old guy to London and all he wants to do is play on these damn escalators!*

On this same day we went to the open air market, bought stuff we wanted but didn't need, then visited the Tower of London, after which we we went to a pub where I enjoyed an authentic Guinness.

This night we had another formal affair, the welcome dinner by our English hosts. The food was as good as the congenial, welcoming manner of the sponsors.

The London Ballroom

It's D Day—D for Dance, Saturday, October 13. We were in the ballroom warming up by 9:00 a.m. for the big day, the reason we came to London! When the event first started it reminded me of a track meet because they called each part a "heat." And the heats came in rapid succession until the early afternoon lunch break, then more dancing until about 7:00 that evening.

Arthur Murray Folsom was noticed, as we were probably the most enthusiastic and vocal, with our cheering and dance moves on the sideline to support the performing dancers, English and American. Our sister Arthur Murray studio from Carmichael, CA, (pronounced Car-mishel by our English hosts) was also there in full force.

I was impressed by the performances of my fellow students, Rustin, Gail and Deanna. They all started lessons just a few months ago, but knew more dances, and did them better than I; or so it seemed to me.

One surprise was the relatively low number of participants. Our host explained that, unlike most years, the folks from the Continent didn't come because their currency had such a low value. The Euro? I didn't quite understand that. Perhaps a boycott against Brexit?

There were a lot of English as well as Americans who performed marvelously. Some of the students seemed to me of professional level. It made me wonder: *What am I doing here?* But that didn't deter me; I went ahead and had fun, did my thirty dances, some well, and others not so well. I originally thought that thirty dances sounded like a lot, but when I found out that my colleagues did as many as sixty, I realized my itinerary was wimpy by comparison.

The Solos

We all had at least one solo to do. It's always a little nerve wracking when just you and your partner are the only ones in the middle of this ballroom floor performing before the rest of the world as you know it right then. In anticipation our nerves tingle and we wonder: How soon can I do my solo and get it over with? This day all solos came at the very end of the day, not until 6:00 p.m. Nice. That gave us plenty of time to fret and build up the tension. But when the time came I wasn't as nervous as usual. Besides, Kate and I felt like we knew our routine pretty well, we had been dancing all day and I told myself this was just another dance.

So finally . . . Kate and I took our place and heard the announcement: "Harvey and his teacher, Kate, from Arthur Murray Folsom, to do the . . . POLKA!"

It went fast and I wasn't aware of any mistakes. When I saw the judge's scores after returning home I found out we got a gold rating for our routine. YAY! It looked to me like all of our team did quite well.

After the solos they had a cocktail hour, serving wine and champagne only, no beer. Maybe I should try to develop a taste for something besides beer, but nothing matches the flavor of hops if that's what you're used to. But that was not the real problem.

Cocktail Hour and Another Wonderful, Formal

Dinner

The cocktail hour was awkward for me, not for the lack of beer, but because I couldn't recognize these people I had been looking at all day at the dance venue. The judges across the dance floor, the organizers, announcers, and the dancers who came out multiple times. Beyond a foot or two they were just forms, anonymous sticks, for me not individually identifiable.

Therefore when I saw these same people close up, I had no idea who anyone was. I would liked to have asked them questions about judging, complimented them on their routines, asked where the name "Barnett," a section of London, came from because that's my middle name. But instead I just stood there looking around, listening and wondering who was who. However, I guess that if this was the worst experience I had in London, I was very lucky, so I'll shuck it off as inconsequential.

From there were treated to a gourmet multi-course dinner. Afterward each group was called up so we could meet all the judges and hosts individually, and each of us was presented with a beautiful *Participation Trophy*. I told my group I was going tell the folks at my senior community that my trophy was for getting first place in the entire event.

Sunday, October 14. I wanted to explore Hyde Park which was only two blocks from our hotel. I yearned to get into nature as well as do some people-watching. Rustin graciously agreed to walk over there with me. On arriving we saw runners with numbers, and crowds lined up on the course cheering them on. It was a Half Marathon, and the runners came and flowed forever, like an unending river. A supporter, with that typical British intonation yelled to the runners, "Yi're amaai-zing!, So I echoed, yelling "Absolutely Amaai-zing!" He turned to me and yelled back, "Incredible!"

So now when someone asks, "How was London?" I answer with my British accent, "Absolutely amaai-zing!

Later, several of us went to the pub named *The Three Tuns* for lunch. I was curious about the word *tun* and learned it is: "*Old English, unit of liquid volume (not weight), used for measuring wine, oil or honey.*" (Or in my case, beer: "I'll have two tuns of your best Guinness then!"

To make the most of this last day in London, Gail, always resourceful, researched live theater and got tickets for *Matilda,* a top notch musical. It was the caliber of a New York Broadway musical and I felt fortunate to be watching this spectacle. I could hear Wesley chuckling appreciatively, relating closely to the scenes because he himself had previously been involved in this same production in another city.

After we left the theater I was ready to sup, so my friends let me pick the pub, which was *The White Lion.* Their Shepard's Pie was excellent. I now had a much better impression of English food.

Monday—another ten hour flight to get home. It was nearly as tolerable as the flight coming over, but the jet lag afterward at home kept kicking me in the patootee for over two weeks. It seemed to mimic the affliction called *chronic fatigue syndrome* that plagues some unfortunates and I empathized with then. But it was well worth it, and now I'm good again, and thankful for the experience.

Chapter Twenty-Five
Empty Nest Ruffled

Of course my son and his wife miss their children who are both in college now, big girls, doing their own thing. The parents love their daughters and look forward to their visits, but meanwhile Mom and Dad have more freedom to spend time doing what they want to do. No more back-to-school nights, volleyball games to attend or coach, theatrical performances, track meets or choir performances. Not that they minded, but sometimes it seemed like they lived their life for their kids! They knew it was worth it, but after all that dedication they've earned the right to live their own life again.

But, alas, recently, there have been new requests coming from another direction. They now have to listen to demands, albeit subtle, from a different quarter; an unlikely one at that.

Wife Tresa: "Oh, we'd love to join you, but we have a . . . conflict that night."

Friend: "Really? What's going on?"

Tresa: "We have to go to a . . . like a dance recital."

Friend: "A dance recital! I thought all your kids were in college."

Will: "It's my eighty-nine year old dad. He's started dance lessons, and is so involved that he's performing at the Arthur Murray Folsom studio Friday night. Just him and his teacher are doing a routine they've been working on. So . . . we feel like we should support him. And he wants us to get a video of his routine."

Friend: "How about your sister? Can't she fill in that night?

Will: "Julie? No, not this time. She told me that Friday night at 8:30 is about the time she's getting ready to go to bed, not drive all the way from West Sacramento to Folsom at night! She'll go to his next daytime dance event, she said."

And she has done so happily several times. All my kids are actually very supportive and come whenever they can.

I do feel a little guilty though, that I'm disrupting their empty nest leisure time. They can't send me off to college, and I'm darn sure not going to get a job.

But at least they don't have to spoon-feed me, or visit me in a nursing home, or run me to the doctor every other day. Besides, when I do have a doctor's appointment I walk there.

The Spotlight Dance

It was billed as *THE GREATEST SHOWMAN SPOTLIGHT PARTY*.

I was not the *Greatest Showman*, I was the *Strong man*. Anyway, that was the role I was playing for my solo routine. This was all my teacher Brandi's idea; I'm not exactly sure why I was to be so strong, except that recently I was doing an aggressive polka spin with Zoila and she exclaimed to all present, "Harvey is so strong!"

To make the *strong* aspect more believable, Brandi had outfitted me with a flesh colored muscle shirt which I had fitted on to my slender, one hundred and thirty pound octogenarian frame. This mode of dress in itself caused a few flurries of stares and kidding, like "Wow, I see you have really been working out, yeah!" And "Oh, man, ha, well I won't even ask!"

I almost made a not so grand opening of my act. Seated at my table I heard my event announced, so I stood and started for the dance floor without noticing that the cord of my shoe bag on the floor was wrapped around my ankle and I was dragging the bag with each step. Then I felt it and a friend helped me extricate myself so I avoided falling on my face as I made my grand entrance on to the ballroom floor.

I had agreed to do this solo routine because it would be a challenge. It was also nerve-wracking. I felt vaguely like I used to before a football game when I was in high school. *What if I drop a pass? What if I miss a key tackle?* Too many *what-ifs*.

Or like the sensation I had before a cross country ski race. Nothing to get nervous about there, though, except maybe a face plant if you lose a ski edge on that downhill curve, but that's not likely. It's mainly a matter of stamina and fitness.

But a dance routine is different. There are so many precise patterns, you and your partner always have to be in sync, and everyone else in the ballroom is watching just the two of you.

The dance I was about to do was fast paced with quick transitions between moves. Could I link up all those transitions properly?

Before the actual dancing part of the routine I did my *strong man* act, flexing my mighty, fake muscles, then hefting a huge *imaginary* barbell to impress the audience. Then Brandi and I came together into dance position and started an energetic Lindy hop. It went fast, and fortunately fairly seamless. A couple of basic patterns with turns a waist roll, link, the jig, the Charleston, sweetheart, walks-and-points, her rollout, my rollout, holding her for her dip and the finale with both of us simultaneously shooting an arm up and yelling a hearty, "YEAH!"

For me the shouting expressed not only exhilaration but also relief that it was over without any major mistakes. And I would have known, for the performers always know if they mess up, even if the spectators don't. The dance goddesses were good to me that day.

There was a lunch break, but the rest of the time there was steady dancing, heat after heat.

I watched my contemporaries doing cha chas, Salsas and rhumbas with moves I'd never heard of, the ladies spinning their legs so fast they became invisible. I saw tangos that transported me to Buenos Aires, if only momentarily. There were swing dances that made me feel like I was watching *Saturday Night Fever* or *Happy Feet* at the movies.

Most of these were students with their teachers, but done so brilliantly that once more I asked myself— *what am I doing here amidst all these super dancers?* But I quickly returned to enjoy the moment. During some of the performances, many of us lined the dance floor for some rhythmic gyrating while we cheered on the performers who were doing their routines.

We had been there since 9:40 in the morning and now it was after 6:00 and time to head home. And so, this, my friends, is what you can look forward to if you go to an Arthur Murray Spotlight Party. You won't know until you try it!

Chapter Twenty-Six
How Dancing Has Enhanced My Life

Alternative Social Settings

It is 9:35 on a Wednesday night as I enter my residence. "Hello, Harvey," the concierge greets me. "Out dancing again?"

"Yep."

One hundred and twenty people live here, but it is as quiet as my family home was at 2:30 a.m. when I was a teenager sneaking into my house and trying not to wake up my parents.

But here, all the inmates, as we sometimes refer to ourselves, are securely ensconced in their cells— that is, apartments. I reside in a senior housing complex, or what I've been calling *The old Folks Home*. I'm lucky to be here because there are amenities and a lot of nice people whose company I enjoy. We have certain things in common, like heart disease, arthritis, high blood pressure, side effects of prescriptions, and hemorrhoids, but we don't discuss the latter.

But sometimes I feel like I am a mobile, rough edged, piece of wood trying to fit into an aperture that is designed for more rounded, smooth and inert tenants.

So I pursue several *out-of-house* interests. At the gym I mix with a bunch of young hard-bodies whose presence give me a boost, but that doesn't mean I try to keep up with them.

I am fortunate to see my kids, grandkids, and great grandkids often. I still have a few friends I get together with once in a while.

But then comes Monday, what used to be a dead day. But nowadays I don't get bored, because I have my dance lesson that afternoon. Then comes a formerly dull Wednesday and there's a dance that night. And there's another one Friday night, if I choose to go, and another on Saturday afternoon as well.

My co-residents here see me going and coming at all hours. "He's always going somewhere," I hear a lady whisper as I head for the exit.

But on St. Patrick's Day I brought the entertainment here to my old folks' home. It was only with the help of my wonderful dance partners that I was able to provide Irish dancing that day. The lovely elders here were clapping with appreciation to the rousing music of our finale.

Help Promoting My Book

One night at a Wednesday night dance party, Kate Gonzalez, the Arthur Murray Folsom Franchise owner, announced the publication of the book I had just finished, titled *Surviving the Old Folks Home*. It was about my experience living in senior communities. Later the dance center sponsored a book signing for me at a practice party. The Arthur Murray staff also performed a hilarious skit, with instructor Brandi reading passages from my book as the others acted out the scenes.

I signed and sold many books that night.

Birthday Celebration

When I turned ninety in August of 2019, Arthur Murray Folsom helped me celebrate it— big time.

The moment I entered the studio for this Friday night dance party, I was greeted with numerous hugs, birthday wishes, and photo requests, then a crown was placed on my head with the number ninety, which I was to wear all evening.

Later they had the traditional birthday dance. My first partner was my teacher, just the two of us on the floor, then my partners rotated, one lady after another. It is the first time I've ever had women lining up to dance with me.

There was also a polka played in my honor, so I danced again, and eventually a young girl stepped in to polka with me. The announcer said, "How many years do you suppose separate these two dancers?" The answer was seventy-eight. Yep, a tender twelve year old and a gnarled ninety year old, the two extremes.

The ballroom was well decorated, with a big numeral ninety on the wall above a table that held cakes and a homemade apple pie, my favorite dessert, baked by my friend, Gail. I had a piece for breakfast the following morning.

There was also the happy birthday song, then I had to blow out the candles on three cakes.

This amazing evening would never have taken place, had I not stepped out of my comfort zone and into dancing.

Return to Polka Land

I had been yearning to get back to the *Polka Boosters Club* that I had belonged to years ago, but had no way to get there and no-one to go with. But after getting acquainted with several nice people at the dance center, I persuaded the most adventurous of them to check out a real polka event. It was a boisterous but friendly atmosphere and it gave me a chance to clarify that when I yell out while dancing the polka at Arthur Murray, it's not me going crazy, it's just what you do at a polka. It is a happy dance.

Special Festivities

Because of my dancing activities at Arthur Murray, I was able to pay visits to the western swing scene with a partner. But even more amazing was the opportunity to go to London.

And then there was the very special dinner dance at Christmas time with a live band in the ballroom of a big hotel. I felt at home there with all my dance friends as we did the cha cha, salsa, hustle, and more.

Fashion Show

I had never before seen a fashion show but I was invited to this one to perform. The location was Old Folsom, and the theme was the fashions of the 1920s. I was born in that decade, so my presence there wasn't inappropriate. Besides, Kate asked me to come and she has treated me well at Arthur Murray, so how could I turn her down?

Gail, who was my partner, looked very chic and young in her snazzy flapper costume. I was just in a suit, but it was so old it probably looked like it came from the 1920s. High schoolers Chris and Faith were the other Arthur Murray students performing this day. They danced the Lindy hop and the Charleston. They were *incredible!* It was tough for Gail and I to follow such a quality performance, but nonetheless we did our rhumba and foxtrot and the audience seemed to appreciate our efforts too.

To have a "surprise ending," coordinator Ronit instructed Gail to stop half way through the foxtrot, and bring young Faith on to dance with me. Then, instead of continuing the fox trop I led her into the Lindy hop. Great fun!

But our dances were just a fill in, the fashion show went on the rest of the time. You should have seen all those old dresses and other garb of the early 1900s! The narrator described the time and circumstances that went went with the mode of dress. At one point the *flapper girls* were featured, in full costume, sashaying in, as the narrator explained, ". . . and these ladies smoked and drank," and then the cops blasted in and chased these lawbreaking girls.

I expected a fashion show to be dull, but this was rather entertaining and quite well managed. Kudos to the organizers!

Friendships

Psychologists, social workers and other authorities say that making new friends is one way to stay happy and well balanced. As we age, we often lose track of current friends and it's not easy to make new ones, so how do we do that? There are at least two elements that are necessary if you're going to make a solid friendship.

Consistency is one requirement for a healthy relationship. Without regularity, it is not likely to endure. The key to making friends as adults is in making time in your week to get together with your new acquaintances to allow those relationships to grow.

Commonality is also a huge foundation of friendship. There needs to be at least one thing that both you and your prospective new friend can relate to, or an activity that you both enjoy.

Don't the above requirements for making new friends describe a dance venue?

Here is a typical dance scenario which I observed: I had come to a dance party with a very nice couple who had graciously invited me to come with them, having heard of my non-driving status. After the music stopped and then we heard, "Thanks for coming," by the DJ, I assumed it was time to leave. I had changed my shoes and was ready. *Where are the people I came with?* I wondered. Then I saw them, standing with a group of people, talking. They didn't look like they were going anyplace. *What's going on?* Then I noticed that no one looked like they were in a hurry to leave. They were all standing around, couples and groups, just happily socializing.

As I observed, I ruminated. *This looks more like a reunion of friends or family, not just a dance.* Then it hit me: All these folks met and became friends. There it is again: regularity and compatibility. Dancing is a natural mixer.

I heard a feminine voice. "Harvey, if you need a ride, I can pick you up, I don't live that far away." It was one of my dance partners; eventually a few others made the same offer, just because they wanted to help a new friend.

Now I linger for a few minutes or more after a dance, the same as I saw the folks doing that other time. I have made many friends at Arthur Murray Folsom. Most of them are much younger than I, but it doesn't matter because we are all centered on dancing.

Some folks who got acquainted at the dance venue have found other common interests besides dancing, such as hiking, traveling, skiing, theater, or concerts.

Interesting things happen when you are consistently in the same place with apparent strangers. Here is what happened after the book signing when I had explained that I used to go by the name Barney.

"So . . . you're the same Barney Jones, who taught at at Del Campo High School at the same time that we were teaching there."

This was a couple I had taught with, but after some twenty-five years we hadn't recognized each other. As we brought up memories about our former teaching colleagues, we changed from casual acquaintances to friends, and thereafter even shared a couple of social occasions.

I was also privileged to go on a hike with some of the other dance friends, as well as some off-site dance events. Maybe the heading for this part should have been: *How to make friends while you kick up your heels.*

The Happy Place

One day I noticed that one of my dance partners, I'll call her April, looked subdued, her usual smile missing. When I inquired, she admitted that her sadness was a result of several recent deaths in her family, one after the other. I was afraid she would be too despondent to return to the dance studio.

But the next week she was back. "My therapist said it's not good to spend time alone, but to find places and people that are upbeat and friendly. I immediately thought, what better place than here? It's the happiest place I know of!"

I'm sure that April still thinks about her late family members from time to time, but during the following weeks her smile returned and she became beautiful again.

The next time it was my turn. My oldest son was racked with two awful diseases. He remained mostly comatose so my family and I had made the awful decision to remove all his life-support systems. This was done the same day I had a dance lesson.

"Hi Harvey!" Brandi greeted me as I entered the studio, "How are you?"

I could only shake my head. "I can't talk," I answered. "Let's just dance."

That Friday night, following the same common sense advice that April's therapist had given her, I came to the practice dance. I was not in good shape emotionally, but the dancing distracted me enough to get some relief. Afterwards, a few people, including April, gathered around me in support. I blubbered a little, but felt reinforced by the empathetic force surrounding me. The dance was over, but teacher Ronit said, "C'mon dance with me." So we danced and she said, "I know you like to sing, so sing me a song."

So I sang. She laughed at the lyrics. My spirits rose with her laughter and the knowledge that I was in a caring place. It might not be easy, but I knew then that I would make it through this ordeal.

Teacher Zoila said it the best: "People come in here and we teach them to dance and help them. Sometimes they're not happy when they come in. But by the time they leave—they're always happy."

Posture

I feel like there is an elastic cord running the length of my body, and its default position is set to make my head slump down and my back curve.

I've gotten so used to that faulty default position of my elastic cord that it is my most comfortable stance. In order to stand erect with my chin tucked a bit (keep your head over your heart) like I'm supposed to requires a conscious effort because it doesn't feel natural. That's because the muscles I use for good posture have gotten so lazy.

But fortunately I am capable of assuming a good posture when it's a conscious act. Some people are not able to straighten up after years of slouching because it has caused spinal misalignment, so they walk around in the shape of a C, bent and staring down at the floor—because that takes the least effort and is more comfortable.

It's like the husband who is habitually slumped on the couch while his wife is working in the kitchen. He tells her, as he takes another pull on his beer, "Ya know, hon, you are the apple of my eye."

And she replies, "Yes, and you are the potato of my couch."

This image of the couch sloucher is what comes to mind when I realize I'm slouching. I equate it with the good posture muscles slouching lazily. I'm afraid that if I spend to much time in that comfortable position, my bent back may freeze in place.

Comfort can be a good thing, but it cannot have first priority in activities such as skiing, hiking, climbing, dancing, or even while standing or walking. But if

you've trained your muscles to be comfortable with good posture, you don't have to worry about this stuff—like I do.

Because of dancing I have become more conscious of my posture than ever before. This has been reinforced by the trainer at the gym, who told me, "Tuck your chin and keep a straight back."

But you won't be able to use me as a model because after so many decades of a comfortable slump, my bearing is far from that of a trained dancer or a young athlete; but everyday while walking or standing I stretch that damned elastic cord out of its default attitude in hopes that it will get used to the new normal. If I can just live that long.

Exercise

The other octogenarian at our dance center said to me one day, "It's good that we're dancing at our age. It's great exercise and it gets us away from that easy chair and TV. Otherwise I'd probably just be sitting around getting lazy."

I agreed. But this is not only relevant for us old retired people, it's applicable across the board. One guest night I was in a group class along with an affable middle aged couple. They were enthusiastic, but both were overweight and looked like our typical *American Sofa Spuds* whose only regular exercise is walking into the kitchen to see what is in the fridge.

They reminded me of what my hiking group called *civilians,* meaning they were inexperienced and clueless about what it takes to enjoy the activity they were about to pursue.

The dance being taught that night was not a fast one; perhaps it was the fox trot or a waltz. The room, as usual, was cool and I was shivering because the moves we were learning were not enough to keep me warm.

After a couple of easy dance patterns, the lady of the couple, obviously out of breath, stopped dancing. "Oh, my goodness, it looks so easy, but doing it is wearing me out! It's more tiring than I thought it would be. I have to sit down." I never saw that couple again.

When I first started dancing I scoffed when friends commented that it was surely good exercise. But I downplayed that contention, saying that the brain got the exercise. That is true, but I was wrong in discounting the physical exercise. I know more dance styles now and admit that two hours of steady dancing is a bona fide workout. As a result I have had to modify my gym days to allow for this additional strenuous activity. And that's okay. Dancing is more fun.

So don't let any gym rat tell you that dancing is not good exercise!

Avoiding Alzheimer's

I've already mentioned that research has shown that ballroom dancing can help prevent Alzheimer's disease because dancing involves different brain functions at the same time.

I'd like to say that I've become brilliant after three years of dance lessons. How nice it would be to claim I can now work out complicated mathematical equations and have learned another foreign language. But this is real life. The goal is to *prevent* Alzheimer's and dementia. Like your muscles, your brain needs constant exercise.

In the senior complex where I live, I see elders my age with varying degrees of memory loss. I also note that many are accustomed to a sedentary life style and lots of TV.

I have had the opportunity to spend time with friends or relatives who were suffering from dementia. What I observed is that the less mental stimulation they had, the faster the disease progressed.

I admit that, like many of my contemporaries. I have been having more trouble than before remembering words and names, and that concerns me. But I have also talked to younger people who say they have the same problem. And besides, I am able to take care of my own finances online, pay my bills, manage my numerous medications, and keep my appointments. I walk to the gym, have to find an unoccupied locker, note the number and location out of over a hundred, and punch in a code. After working out for two or three hours I have to find my locker and remember the code.

On many occasions I couldn't help but observe that some of those young guys had to call in an employee to help them find or open their locker because they forgot which one it was, or hadn't entered the code correctly. I smiled and felt a bit smug.

When I get home and record my workout log, I have no trouble remembering which exercises, which machines I did, including my heart rates for the aerobics. All it takes is concentrating and paying attention.

So I will continue to take ballroom dance lessons to keep my gray matter stimulated and the body parts moving until my nonagenarian systems signal me that I am old. But I may ignore that because I still plan to *live fast and die young.*

Improved Wardrobe

Dressing better boosts your confidence, improves the way you look, and sets you apart as a guy who "gets it."

But I didn't "get it." If you were to look in my closet (please don't), you would be shocked to see such threadbare, outmoded apparel. Some are so out-of-date they come back into fashion. Seeing them would probably make you believe that you were looking into a closet that had been used by some poor bloke now long dead. If I had a wife she would have long ago thrown out three-fourths of these frumpy duds.

Well, I haven't expired, but I sure as hell am old, I figured, so why do I need to put out good money for threads that are supposed to make me look cool? Is it even possible for people this old to look cool? And does it really matter?

When I went to London to dance, I was wearing an old belt that I'd had for years that I had purchased at a thrift store. Evidently it was so bad that my dance partner was motivated to buy me a new one. So maybe it does matter.

After I retired I bought hardly any new clothing and the few new items I bought were either casual or for mountaineering, strictly utilitarian. Any big bucks I parted with were for practical items like Gore Tex jackets with fabric that was both waterproof and breathable; or for those snazzy plastic ski boots. But on my ski outings I wore the same old woolen slacks I had bought thirty years before when I was teaching.

But now I go to dances and big events like the Spotlight Showcase and some formal occasions. This is a new situation that I had not imagined I would be in at this advanced age. I'm not complaining, but my dance instructors dress so stylishly that, by comparison, my apparel makes me look like I might be a homeless character who just wandered in from an encampment.

And how about some of the gowns the ladies wear at the special balls. They are so classy that I hesitate to be in the same room with them because the contrast is so great.

So in my new setting, I have started to upgrade my wardrobe. I'll get some slim-fit pants that don't need altering, find shirts that actually fit me instead of just making do with what I find on the racks. I may not attain *cool,* but I hope that at least I can look like I fit in with this authentically cool crowd.

For my ninetieth birthday I asked my daughter to take me shopping at H & M, where they have all sizes. I made some good clothing purchases, but I still need more. I'm going to have to prevail upon my sweet daughter to take me again. She doesn't know this yet.

Epilogue

Well, now you know all the advantages that go with dancing; such as exercise for body and brain, social benefits and making friends, posture improvement, and adding more variety to your life.

But would you believe dancing can save a marriage?

I admit, at first I was skeptical about this story. But my buddy, Monte, swore this is really how it went down with his friend Peter. Here's the scenario as he described it to me:

Peter had been married with this woman for thirty years and she had fairly recently become so negative that they could hardly have a cordial conversation anymore. He said Peter is about fifty-three and his wife is fifty-one.

"It seems like she's crabby all the time," Peter had told Monte. "She blames it on her period."

"Well, that should only last a very few days each month then," I pointed out. (Not that I'm any expert in this area.)

"Nah, he said her period lasts for two weeks."

"That's abnormally long, isn't it?

"And she has two periods a month!"

"Oh, c'mon," I protested, "that's ridiculous!"

"Peter swears it's true and it's about to wreck his marriage!"

"Okay," I said, "he has to do something special with her. Take her mind off of her troubles."

"Like what?"

"Woo her a little first, then suggest that it would be nice to have dance lessons, just the two of them."

Monte passed this advice on to Peter, who was so desperate that he was ready to try anything. So here's how he said it went with harried husband, Peter, and his perpetual period spouse:

"Hey, hon, how about we go out and scuff the parquet a bit?"

"WHAT?!"

"You know, trip the light fantastic! We could really cut a wicked rug!"

"You mean . . . dance?"

"Yeah, we could take lessons together. It's good exercise and it will get us out of the house."

"Sounds like a stupid idea, but I suppose I'll give it a try if it will shut you up."

After three months of dance lessons the wife's personality changed dramatically. She became a happy person, positive and outgoing, like she had been when Peter first met her.

"It's a miracle!" Peter exclaimed. "And it's cheaper than marriage counseling. But my mother-in-law thinks it's probably just because my wife went into menopause."

But we know better, don't we?

IT WAS THE DANCING!